The Other Side of ADHD

The Other Side of ADHD

Attention deficit hyperactivity disorder exposed and explained

ANGELA SOUTHALL

Head of Specialist Children's Services
South Staffordshire Healthcare NHS Trust

Radcliffe Publishing
Oxford • New York

07/08

Radcliffe Publishing Ltd
18 Marcham Road
Abingdon
Oxon OX14 1AA
United Kingdom

www.radcliffe-oxford.com
Electronic catalogue and worldwide online ordering facility.

British Library Cataloguing in Publication Data

A catalogue record for this book is available from the British Library.

ISBN-13: 978 1 84619 068 1

Typeset by Egan Reid, Auckland, New Zealand
Printed and bound by TJI Digital, Padstow, Cornwall, UK

Contents

For James

About the author

Angela Southall has been working with children, young people and families in an NHS setting since 1986. Since qualifying as a clinical psychologist she has worked tirelessly to promote a psycho-social understanding of children's mental health. Her approach to service delivery has been shaped by her experiences of the problems encountered by children and families in their day-to-day lives. Her commitment to community psychology has led to the initiation and development of a number of multi-agency community services and partnerships, core aspects of which have been the extending of psychological skills to non-specialist practitioners and the inclusion of service users and their families in service design and delivery. Her approach to child and adolescent mental health services has generated new ways of working, as well as demonstrating that it is possible to offer – and sustain – community-based services that are valued and effective, without lengthy periods on 'waiting lists'.

Angela continues to lead a diverse, multi-disciplinary Child Psychology and Psychological Therapies service in Staffordshire, whilst also developing the county's Intensive Fostering Programme, which offers specialist foster care to young offenders as an alternative to custody. This is the first collaborative partnership of its kind between Health, Youth Offending and Family Placement Services.

Angela's clinical specialism is in the field of parenting, attachment and trauma.

Acknowledgements

I am grateful to Abby Marr for additional research and Professor Chris Frith for a very useful conversation that helped my thinking about the brain. Thanks are also due to all of the children, young people and families whom I have met and worked with over the years, without whom none of this would ever have been written. Finally, my thanks to Michael Foulkes for reading the draft manuscript, and for his extremely helpful and encouraging comments.

Author's note

This book contains a number of 'vignettes' which illustrate particular aspects of people's lives and the difficulties that they sometimes encounter. These are composite case histories that bring together some of the characteristics of the kinds of situations and problems that I have come across during the course of my work. None of them describes any single family or individual, but all are nevertheless taken from real–life experiences. Where I have used material sent to me from other professionals in the field, no identifying features have been used.

Introduction: Why I've written this book

This book has been written by a clinician – someone who works with children and families, not someone who just writes about them. I have worked with children for the best part of 20 years. During this time I have seen many ideas come and go. I have heard thousands of stories from families and from individual children and young people. I was asked the other day whether I still find these stories moving, or whether I have just become used to them. The answer was that, yes, I have found myself moved by them, sometimes to tears and sometimes, like now, to action. This book has been motivated by my own day-to-day experiences, not only with children but also with their parents and carers and by those like me who try to help them with their difficulties. It is their experiences that have compelled me to write this book.

Attention deficit hyperactivity disorder (ADHD) has become a clinical phenomenon, a modern-day epidemic of incredible proportions, unlike any we have seen before. Along with thousands of other mental health practitioners, I have watched this state of affairs develop until it has come to affect just about every aspect of children's mental health provision. It has swept over us like a tidal wave.

Over the years I have become aware of more and more children who have this diagnosis. This has created a considerable dilemma for me as a practitioner, because I have found myself in a position where I have been at odds with the prevailing view about these children's problems. As the situation has unfolded, it has seemed to me that the subject of ADHD touches on other important issues, some of which are pivotal to our thinking about mental health. These make ADHD an even more controversial subject than it first appears.

As this condition has 'spread', a great deal of information has been made available, including a number of books. Many of these are excellent and provide a well-reasoned argument for doing things differently. They do not necessarily dispute the dominant story about ADHD, but choose instead to challenge the 'treatment' of so-called 'ADHD children.' Although such literature is no doubt helpful to parents and children, much of it seems to have adopted – remarkably uncritically – the view that ADHD is a bona-fide clinical 'disorder.' The focus is on over-diagnosis, rather than misdiagnosis, and on 'alternative', non-drug treatment. Challenges to the accepted view often seem to focus on one particular aspect of the subject or another, or on the fine detail, leaving the overarching issues more or less undisputed. Few seem to offer an insight into the wider concerns raised by ADHD that help to maintain its current status as probably the most controversial subject in children's mental health.

It is the wider issues that I felt people deserved to know about. It seemed to me that there was a need to pull together the different strands of the debate so that parents and clinicians could build up a more complete picture and make their own informed decisions. I became increasingly concerned that all we were ever hearing in terms of health information was one particular point of view, and I became more and more concerned about why this might be. Outside the professional arena, many of the uncertainties and disagreements around ADHD seemed to remain unheard, including the information, statistics, clinical evidence and real-life stories that suggested to me and many other clinicians that something had gone very wrong.

From 2000, my involvement in ADHD became intense, from both a clinical and a service development perspective. In both cases, the feeling was one of trying to swim against the tide (again, probably not dissimilar to others). At times it felt more akin to drowning. Training others – an important aspect of my job – meant developing my own resources because, although there are some extremely good books and papers out there, trying to develop a more complete story necessitated a search for information that was often obscured or not easily available. I kept waiting for a new story to materialise. There seemed to be hardly any information for families that offered them an opportunity to begin to see the bigger picture. Likewise, few resources existed that would enable students or trainees to develop a comprehensive understanding of ADHD-related issues. This is what prompted me to start collating my own information, an activity that ultimately meant I had no excuse for not writing this book.

This is not a book that offers more information on ADHD, nor is it one whose sole purpose is to challenge the view that ADHD exists (although I hope that through a wider discussion it will help readers to consider this possibility). It is a book that attempts to draw together the issues that ADHD brings into play – clinically, socially, philosophically, ethically and politically.

Chapter 1 begins by discussing ADHD as a diagnostic category, and provides the reader with an overview of some of the key ingredients in the debate regarding its legitimacy as a clinical construct. This raises questions about diagnosis in general and how mental health problems are viewed. The following chapters then discuss the 'treatment of choice' – that is, stimulant medication – and the concerns about drug treatment and its promotion. These chapters lead to an analysis of how the pharmaceutical companies have helped to promote an increasingly biological understanding of mental health problems. Subsequent chapters look at the ways in which our society has changed and the impact that some of these changes have had on children, legitimising psychiatric labels such as ADHD. The book then considers some of the reasons why children have attentional problems, and why it is important to investigate the problems rather than the symptoms. Later chapters examine some of the social and political issues relevant to the debate which suggest that ADHD is not only contentious but also a highly political diagnosis.

This book has another aim – it is intended to take an unashamedly 'one-sided' look at ADHD as a counterbalance to the prevailing view that is expressed in the media. That is, it deliberately sets out to reveal to the reader *the other side of ADHD*. I hope that by doing this, a different kind of debate might be initiated. My best hope is that others will join it and that we might find – together – that the tide is beginning to turn.

CHAPTER 1

What is ADHD?

Attention deficit hyperactivity disorder (ADHD) is a diagnostic term that has been used since 1987 to describe a cluster of behaviours associated with inattention, impulsivity and hyperactivity.* Although the term is used increasingly often, there is widespread disagreement about whether it exists at all and whether it is, in fact, a valid diagnostic category. Although its advocates are prone to describing it in certain terms, there has rarely been so much uncertainty and controversy about a diagnosis that is being used extensively to describe children's behaviour, and which is leading to increases in the prescribing of stimulant medication for children at an unprecedented rate. So high is the degree of concern about the rate of increase in diagnosis and prescribing that enquiries have been initiated in the UK and abroad to try to determine why this is happening.

How are children assessed for ADHD?

There is no single test for ADHD. Most assessments tend to use parent and school reports, combined with 'checklist' data (many assessors use *only* these sources of information). Some (but not all) assessments incorporate additional observational information. After this, a decision is made as to whether or not the child has ADHD.

It will be obvious to any thoughtful reader that this material will be open to inter-pretation. The interpretation, of course, depends on what we might call the assessor's *frame of reference* –the mechanism that they use to understand and interpret what they see. This will have developed over many years and incorporates beliefs, knowledge, prejudices, cultural expectations and experience – it becomes the lens through which they view the world.

In short, ADHD assessment is highly subjective. This is demonstrated by the extreme variation in incidence from country to country and between cities and towns (we shall return to this later in the book). Population data suggest that it is strongly associated with social and psychological factors, such as family income, parental employment status and children's experiences of stressful family life (e.g. parental separation or family breakdown). For many people who work with children and

---

* It replaced the previous category, 'hyperkinetic reaction' (1968).

families, this kind of information adds further impetus to the view that when we give parents and teachers assessment 'checklists', we may not be measuring what we think we are measuring.

Incidence

The past decade has witnessed a remarkably steep increase in the number of children diagnosed with 'ADHD' in Europe and North America. Reported rates of ADHD in school-age children vary, but most estimates lie between 5% and 10%.[1] In the USA, current estimates suggest that as many as 17.8% – *almost one in five schoolchildren* – have this 'disorder.'[2] The trend continues to be an upward one.

In the UK, the figures are lower. Reports suggest a prevalence of between 2% and 5%, depending on which set of diagnostic criteria is applied.[3] Although lower, this figure still equates to *up to one in 20 children*, and will include at least four times as many boys as girls.[4]

Why the increases?

Given these figures, we could be excused for thinking that something strange and unexplained is happening to our children. (After all, this 'disorder' didn't seem to be around earlier, when we were young or when our parents were young. Even 'hyper-activity' did not seem to affect anywhere near as many children.) Therefore we might reason that it must be something to do with modern life. Are modern lifestyles making our children ill?

Or is it just the way we think about children's behaviours nowadays? Are our changed expectations leading us to label some childhood behaviours as problematic, when they might previously have been viewed as normal? Is this the kind of thinking that makes people more likely to look for medical labels for children?

Both of these ideas are important in their own right and have been the subject of much debate among those working with children and families. We shall revisit them later in this book. However, in trying to explain the unprecedented increases in the diagnosis of ADHD and stimulant prescriptions, we need first to look elsewhere. This means focusing on how ADHD has been defined and popularised, and what other factors have been involved in this process.

ADHD as a diagnostic category

The idea of the 'hyperactive' child developed in the 1960s, and it is during this period that the first references to hyperactivity (or *hyperkinesis*) can be found in the *Diagnostic and Statistical Manual (DSM)* published by the American Psychiatric Association.

Originally perceived as a research tool, the *DSM* has developed through a number of revisions into what has often been referred to as the diagnostic 'bible' for mental health. Each new edition has been weightier and has included more and more new diagnoses. The *DSM* has grown longer with each revision (*see* Box 1.1).

BOX 1.1 The growth of the *DSM* since first publication

DSM	1952	100 pages (containing about 60 disorders)
DSM-II	1968	150 pages
DSM-III	1980	500 pages
DSM-III-R	1987	567 pages
DSM-IV	1994	900 pages

On the basis of the above, the *DSM-V*, expected in 2011, has been predicted to have 1,256 pages and to contain 1,800 diagnostic criteria, generating US$ 80 million in revenue for the American Psychiatric Association.[5]

The 1980 edition *(DSM-III)* saw the first appearance of the term 'attention deficit disorder', which significantly expanded the definition of its predecessor, 'hyperkinetic reaction of childhood.' By 1987 (in the *DSM-III-R*), this had become the by now familiar term *attention deficit hyperactivity disorder (ADHD)*. There were still more developments in 1994 with the *DSM-IV*. In this edition, two categories of symptoms are listed, namely 'inattentive' and 'hyperactive/impulsive', and three types of disorder, namely 'ADHD, *primarily inattentive*', 'ADHD, *primarily hyperactive*' and 'ADHD, *combined type.*'

Following the broadening of diagnostic criteria in 1991, the numbers of children diagnosed with ADHD shot up by approximately 60%.[6] In short, definitions of ADHD have come to include more and more children.[7] As a result, ADHD is often held up as an example of 'diagnostic spread', where ever broader definitions of 'disorders' mean that more and more people are caught in the diagnostic 'net.' Critics suggest that categories have now become so wide that we risk labelling normal childhood behaviour 'disordered.'

Decide for yourself. The *DSM-IV* criteria for ADHD are listed in Box 1.2.

BOX 1.2 *DSM-IV* diagnostic criteria for ADHD

A. Either 1 or 2

1. *Six (or more) of the following symptoms of inattention have persisted for at least 6 months to a degree that is maladaptive and inconsistent with developmental level:*
   a. Often fails to give close attention to details or makes careless mistakes in schoolwork or other activities.
   b. Often has difficulty sustaining attention in tasks or play activities.
   c. Often does not listen when spoken to directly.
   d. Often does not follow through on instructions and fails to finish schoolwork, chores or duties in the workplace (not due to oppositional behaviour or failure to understand instructions).
   e. Often has difficulty organising tasks and activities.
   f. Often avoids, dislikes or is reluctant to engage in tasks that require sustained mental effort (such as schoolwork or homework).

cont. overleaf

BOX 1.2 (continued)

    g. Often loses things necessary for tasks and activities (e.g. toys, school assignments, pencils, books or tools).

    h. Is often easily distracted by extraneous stimuli.

    i. Is often forgetful in daily activities.

2. *Six (or more) of the following symptoms of hyperactivity–impulsivity have persisted for at least 6 months to a degree that is maladaptive and inconsistent with developmental level:*

Hyperactivity

    a. Often fidgets with hands or feet, or squirms in seat.

    b. Often leaves seat in classroom or in other situations in which remaining in seat is expected.

    c. Often runs about or climbs excessively in situations in which it is inappropriate (in adolescents or adults, may be limited to subjective feelings of restlessness).

    d. Often has difficulty playing or engaging in leisure activities quietly.

    e. Is often 'on the go' and often acts 'as if driven by a motor.'

    f. Often talks excessively.

Impulsivity

    a. Often blurts out answers before questions have been completed.

    b. Often has difficulty awaiting turn.

    c. Often interrupts or intrudes on others (e.g. butts into conversations or games).

A. Some hyperactive–impulsive or inattentive symptoms that caused impairment were present before 7 years of age.

B. Some impairment from the symptoms is present in two or more settings (e.g. at school or work, or at home).

C. There must be clear evidence of clinically significant impairment in social, academic or occupational functioning.

D. The symptoms do not occur exclusively during the course of a pervasive developmental disorder, schizophrenia or other psychotic disorder, and are not better accounted for by another mental disorder (e.g. mood disorder, anxiety disorder, dissociative disorder or personality disorder).

It is possible, of course, that some readers of this book might have children who do not display these 'symptoms.' If so, I would say they are highly unusual. That is the first problem with this list of behaviours – it describes things that *all* children do. Secondly, there is a reliance on opinion that is rather too subjective. For example, at what stage does 'fidgeting' or 'not listening' – surely very ordinary behaviour in children – reach the clinical threshold? Who decides when something is too much (or not enough)? After all, parents, teachers and doctors vary enormously in what they are prepared to tolerate as 'normal.' The over–inclusiveness of the criteria, together with their reliance on subjectivity, has led to much criticism. Indeed, some have alleged that the criteria are pretty meaningless. Among these critics is psychiatrist Peter Breggin, who suggests that the *DSM* criteria are nothing but lists of behaviours that need more attention from the teacher.[8]

Breggin is one of many children's specialists who have expressed concern. On the face of it, it seems that there is indeed cause for concern. Not just our children but also the adult population seems to be more and more prone to mental illness these days. As we can see by the steady growth of the *DSM*, more disorders are being 'discovered' year on year. Their increasing number and the broadening of some, such as ADHD, make it imperative that we step back and ask ourselves what this kind of mental health classification really means.

How 'real' are diagnostic categories?

It is important to recognise that the system of classification of mental illness was originally set up for research purposes and that it is *subjective*. That is, like any system it is a product of professional, social, cultural and political thinking during a particular period in time. To appreciate this, we only have to remind ourselves that until 1973 homosexuality was still classified as a mental disorder and appeared in the *DSM* under the category of 'sociopathic personality disturbance.' Homosexuals were no different in 1973 than in 1972. They had not suddenly changed their sexual preferences and practices. What *had* changed was the way in which homosexuality was classified, or rather de-classified, reflecting the thinking of the day. Homosexuality is just one of a number of examples that illustrate how judgements about what is or isn't disordered behaviour change according to the view of the day. Diagnostic categories are not 'fixed' entities, nor are they objective realities. They exist only because we invent them. The problem with the *DSM* is that it provides a supposedly expert view and a certainty that just isn't there.

Biological explanation of problem + pharmacological solution = biological problem (or 2 + 2 = 5)

From the time when mental ill health began to be studied, biological explanations have been assumed and acted upon. This has been the thinking that has placed mental health firmly within the domain of medicine. The assumption has been that the same kinds of processes that cause physical health problems also underlie mental health ones, and therefore – so the logic goes – they can be 'cured' in the same way, by medical intervention. This assumption has become so pervasive that it is seen as a 'truth' that is beyond challenge. Richard Bentall, in his book *Madness Explained*, examines in detail these 'truths' – the many assumptions that underpin the biological diagnostic framework.[9] He then considers the evidence relating to them. What emerges is a persuasive and well-reasoned case for leaving behind a diagnostic system that, ironically, cannot withstand reasoned analysis.

How beliefs about mental ill health have changed over the centuries

In the past, 'cures' for mental disorders have involved some fairly horrific practices. In the sixteenth century, if you were deemed 'mad' you stood a chance of being burned, tortured or drowned as a witch or as someone possessed by demons. In the seventeenth century, you might have been isolated along with other 'undesirables', such as the poor and destitute, criminals and those with disabilities. You might have been kept in chains or shackles, or perhaps even in a dungeon. During the eighteenth century you would have found yourself the subject of increasing medical scrutiny, although still kept in degrading and dirty conditions where, for a fee, visitors might be allowed to come and ogle you. In the nineteenth century, you would have been subject to a range of pseudo-medical practices. These included 'bleeding', which consisted of inducing bleeding in the temples or from a vein in the foot, or by using leeches. Other 'cures' included cold baths or plunging the patient into cold water. Long-term treatments with 'purges', which included various methods of inducing vomiting and diarrhoea, were also popular. These methods would often be continued for many years. The fact that the patient did not get better was taken as a sign that the treatment needed to be continued. In the twentieth century, such treatments were superseded by new ones, developed from a psychiatry that now located the seat of insanity in the brain. Medical and surgical methods, such as frontal lobotomies, electric shock treatment and insulin coma, became the new 'cures' (*see* Figure 1.1).

With the 'discovery' (by accident) of psychotropic drugs, drug treatment became the panacea. What followed this discovery is hugely important because its underlying philosophy still applies to twenty-first-century drug treatment – *whatever seemed to 'work' was believed to indicate the underlying problem*. This is still the case.

Modern psychiatry

What has been the progress of psychiatry up to the present day? Surprisingly little, according to some authors. Richard Bentall, reviewing the evidence, concludes that few improvements have been made since the beginning of the century, despite the introduction of psychoactive drugs.[10] Drug treatment has not led to the promised 'cures' for mental health problems in our society. Instead, we have a situation where more and more drugs are discovered and promoted year on year, accompanied by a corresponding increase in the number of people classified as having mental health disorders. We are told that one in four people will experience some kind of mental health problem in the course of a year, while 20% of women and 14% of men in England apparently have some form of mental illness.[11]

While time has marched forward, the fundamental assumptions underlying psychiatric diagnosis and treatment have not changed. The same ideas underlie the bottle of antidepressants or stimulants as treatment by purging, brain surgery and electroconvulsive therapy (electric shock treatment). The assumption is this – you feel and behave the way you do because *there is something wrong with your brain*.

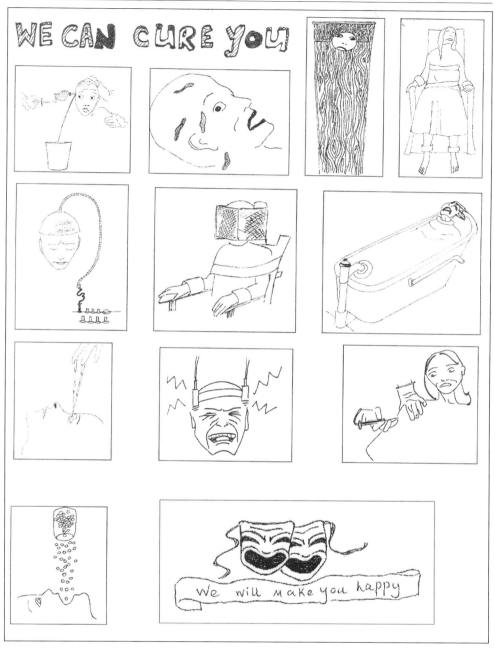

FIGURE 1.1 'We can cure you.'

The psychosocial model and 'talking therapies'

Since the middle of the twentieth century there have been considerable developments in mental health knowledge. Some of these have been reflected in therapeutic practice through a range of psychological therapies, as well as in the theoretical understanding that underpins it. These relate to the *psychosocial* model of mental health (*see* Box 1.3). The changes in thinking and present-day understanding about the family and the environmental, social, educational and cultural factors that contribute to mental health problems make it difficult for many practitioners to match their learning and experience with the kind of medical classificatory system that still prevails and which is exemplified by the *DSM*.

BOX 1.3 The psychosocial model of mental health

The psychosocial model of mental health was developed in the 1960s in direct opposition to the dominant philosophy of the time, which was, of course, medical. Psychosocial approaches emphasise the importance of the social and relational context in which we live. Psychological well-being is determined by these contexts, as well as the psychological processes that underlie human development and behaviour. It is this *interaction* between our life events and our underlying psychological processes that determines whether or not we are able to cope with life and the many adversities it presents us with. This is the complex 'mental health' equation that explains how the balance can be tipped for any one of us. The possibility of emotional ill-health exists for us all: it simply requires the right set of circumstances.

For some years now there has been increasing dissent within the mental health field, with a growing number of psychologists, psychotherapists and psychiatrists suggesting that people do not fit into the kinds of categories contained within the *DSM*. Some clinicians and therapists have suggested that such 'labelling' is so misleading that it serves no useful purpose and should be abandoned altogether. They argue that the life experiences of people with mental health difficulties make their distress wholly understandable and explainable according to their family circumstances, past experiences and current resources. Explaining away such difficulties by locating the problem in their brain is not that far removed from the old ideas of possession – it removes the problem from everyone else and locates it firmly within the individual.

It is difficult to imagine how a diagnostic system that does all of these things, that is so subjective that it creates new disorders and removes others at will, and still seeks to categorise human behaviour – in all its complexity – in keeping with long-abandoned beliefs, can maintain its credibility. How can this be the case?

Systems of classification

Basically, systems of classification are whatever we want them to be. How enduring and influential they are and the extent to which they are adopted by society are probably determined by whether or not they are useful to those in power, not by whether they are 'real' – they can never be real.

The *DSM* has at its foundation a set of ideas based on an outdated system. A good parallel would be something like the *Ptolemaic system* of the universe. Think about it for a moment. This, too, was an elegant and detailed classificatory system, one that was based on the idea of the earth being at the centre of the universe, and the sun and other planets moving around it in perfect synchronicity. The Christianised Ptolemaic system is exemplified by Dante's poem, *The Divine Comedy*, in which he describes a journey through hell, purgatory and paradise. Dante's universe was a divinely ordered hierarchy within which all creatures, including angels, obeyed divine laws and were subject to detailed classification. As classification systems go, this would probably take the prize for the most detailed, all-encompassing one of all time. It was enduring because it suited the purpose of the church at that time. The Ptolemaic system existed, more or less unchanged and unchallenged, for over 1000 years until Galileo Galilei reported his findings in the early part of the seventeenth century (*see* Box 1.4). And what is the moral of this story? Just because something seems like the established truth and is elegantly worked out and articulated, that doesn't necessarily make it right.

BOX 1.4 Galileo's challenge to the system

In 1609, Galileo first pointed his telescope towards the moon. After this, he began to make discoveries about the planets and their movements which contradicted Ptolemy's model of the universe – where all heavenly bodies were believed to be attached to crystal spheres that rotated around the earth in perfect synchronicity. This brought Galileo into conflict with the Catholic Church. Following the publication of his theories in 1632, the Inquisition found him guilty of heresy. Although the evidence was there to enable church scholars to see for themselves that the existing classificatory system could not possibly be correct, they refused to consider it. It presented too much of a challenge to the belief system that had been established and upon which the prevailing theories and 'truths' of the day appeared to rest.

The *DSM*, like the Ptolemaic system before it, lays claim to foundations that are solidly embedded within science – this lends it an undeserved respectability and credibility, and has made it so much a part of modern-day psychiatry that it has become a strong thread running through all of our thinking about mental health difficulties. This is a process otherwise known as 'hegemony' – the means by which particular systems of values, attitudes and beliefs combine to become the established and accepted way of viewing the world. The 'world view' is developed, supported and maintained by those who have power and control, and it becomes an integral part of every aspect of people's lives. It is so pervasive that it is accepted as the only sensible way of seeing things. It becomes unchallengeable.

This is the spirit in which ADHD has been received and acted upon. But mental health should involve more than just an act of faith. It should be about developing knowledge through rigorous examination of fact and then using this knowledge to develop new approaches to helping, based on evidence of effectiveness. Evidence should be unequivocal – that is, it must be indisputable. Otherwise how can we possibly claim that anything 'works'?

What happens if we apply these criteria to ADHD? Let's look at some of the evidence.

ADHD as a biological disorder

In keeping with the biological explanation, ADHD is assumed to have a neurobiological or neurochemical basis. However, despite extensive research over almost 30 years, there is still no unequivocal evidence to this effect. It remains only a hypothesis – a theory. In fact, in 1998 the American National Institutes of Health took the step of announcing that there was *no evidence that ADHD was a biological brain disorder*. This position remains unchanged.

The search for genetic links

Statements about ADHD as a biological disorder are often followed by claims of genetic relationships. In establishing the credibility of ADHD's supposedly biological status, it is important to be able to prove that it is 'inherited.' However, although there continue to be many claims that ADHD has a genetic link, this also remains unproven.

BOX 1.5 The great nature/nurture debate

The 'nature/nurture' issue is at the centre of one of the longest running debates in psychology. Is human development the result of our genetic inheritance or of the influence of environment°? This question has been applied to a number of areas, notably mental illness, intelligence and criminality. Despite decades of research, the evidence continues to suggest that it is the quality of our lives – 'nurture' – that is most important in determining psychological well-being, whatever the problem. Psychotic illnesses such as 'schizophrenia' have been extensively studied and are probably best known for having a reputed genetic basis. This, too, does not stand up to scrutiny. When the evidence is examined, inheritance seems to be only one of many complex factors that interact together. Above all, it is the quality and type of experiences we have in our various family environments that play the greater part in determining who we are. Shared experiences, rather than shared genes, determine similarities in family networks.[12] All in all, it seems, as Lewis and colleagues told us in 2000, that 'the genetic lottery may determine the cards in your deck, but experience deals you the hand you can play . . .'.[13,14]

In general, much theorising about genetic origins of mental illnesses comes from twin studies. As you might expect, a number of these studies have claimed to demonstrate genetic links in ADHD. Many of these are based on twin studies that have compared 'ADHD rates' between identical (monozygotic) and non–identical (dizygotic) twins. The rationale on which such studies are based is that identical twins share more of

---

* The term 'environment' is an inadequate and misleading one. It refers not only to the physical environment of the person but also to its social, emotional and relational qualities, as well as the complex way in which all of these processes interact.

their genetic make-up, which means (so the theory goes) that a higher incidence of ADHD must therefore be evidence of a genetic cause ('nature'), rather than an environmental one ('nurture').

This kind of research is not new to mental health, of course, where there continues to be disagreement about the assumptions made by investigators using twin studies.

So far as the ADHD studies are concerned, although there have been reportedly higher correlations of ADHD between identical twins,[15] critics dispute whether this provides evidence of inheritance. As is the case with twin comparison studies generally, there are a number of problems with the assumptions that they make about 'environment' and what is called 'gene expression' (the influences upon genes, and the way that genes in turn influence behaviour). Basically, critics of twin studies suggest that they oversimplify the complex issue of genetic inheritance.

The problem with twins . . .

One of the most comprehensive reviews of twin studies has been undertaken by Jay Joseph in his book, *The Gene Illusion*.[16] Here Joseph outlines in considerable detail the consistent misinterpretation of findings of twin studies over more than half a century. He presents a powerful argument that twin studies, despite what is commonly believed, are 'unable to disentangle possible genetic influences.' In other words, greater similarities between identical twins are just as likely to be the result of environmental factors as of genetic ones.

Having scrutinised the claims made by twin studies in schizophrenia and found them unsound, Joseph concludes that:

> Like schizophrenia, the evidence supporting the brain disease theory of ADHD is weak. The genetic evidence consists of family studies, twin studies and adoption studies *far more flawed* than their schizophrenia counterparts. (my italics)

Similarly, in 2003, Albert Galves and his colleagues[17] reviewed the claims made by ADHD twin study researchers, and also emphasised their shortcomings. Their paper also points out that environmental factors such as stress, trauma and lack of parental responsiveness have an effect on protein and protein synthesis in genes. Thus the process whereby genes influence the behavioural characteristics of a person is *itself* greatly influenced by environmental factors.

Infant temperament

Other researchers looking at genetic links to ADHD have reported 'infant temperament' as a possible predictor of later ADHD.[18] This is interpreted by some as evidence that the condition is present from birth, and therefore inherited. To anyone who works with young children and knows even a little about child development, such conclusions are quite remarkable in their simplicity. They ignore the importance of the infant's family environment, in particular the relationships between babies, carers and the environments in which they live. Those who draw conclusions about 'inheritance' based on reported infant temperament fail to appreciate the extraordinary importance of relational and environmental factors in all aspects of child development. With similar single-mindedness, comparison studies among relatives, supposedly demonstrating 'proof' of a genetic link, ignore crucial relational, environmental and cultural similarities that are likely to exist across generations.

Given that we all have families, we are all in a position to reflect on some of the 'ingredients' that make us what we are. Despite our very best intentions, parenting practices tend to be repeated, socio-economic status tends to remain fairly static, and family values, beliefs and attitudes remain remarkably constant across generations. These circumstances help to explain why history repeats itself so regularly. It is probably not difficult for us to recall from our own family histories 'things that run in the family.' This is not at all the same as being genetic – in fact, it couldn't be more different.

What's the verdict?

Despite the best efforts of researchers over a considerable period of time, and a significant amount of investment in research, there is still no unequivocal evidence that ADHD is a 'biological disorder', either in terms of inheritance or in terms of 'genes.' Rather, the evidence suggests the opposite – that similarities among family members are just as likely to be the result of important environmental factors. Nevertheless, we continue to pour more and more money into ADHD research in a search for 'proof' of a biological basis. Why do we do this? Well, at least part of the answer must be to do with the fact that there is money to be made in discovering this 'proof', notably by the drug companies who finance much of the research that seeks it. Conversely, there is no profit at all to be made from researching psychosocial aspects of children's problems and non-drug ways of helping them. Just imagine what might be achieved if this money – and effort – could be reinvested.

So the scenario looks set to continue. ADHD research will go on in much the same vein. Despite the weakness of many of the claims, a great deal has been made of the ADHD biological research to date. Some of this has been (erroneously) reported as already having provided proof of biological and genetic links. These claims tend to be highly publicised in the media (in contrast to the retractions and debates that usually follow). The result has been a disaster for healthcare professionals, parents and children alike, as it has produced a climate in which *we think we already know about ADHD.*

The problem of false certainty

The difficulty with some of the ADHD literature is not one of hypothesising – good practice requires that we have ideas about things and check them out. This is the way we make progress in our understanding about people's difficulties and how to help them. No, the problem is not in the ideas – it is one of *false certainty.* As this is being written, there is a multiplicity of leaflets, as well as Internet websites and various other sources of information, that state very clearly and categorically that ADHD is a neurobiological disorder with a strong genetic component, and that the most successful treatment is stimulant medication, usually Ritalin. All of these assertions are nothing more than *beliefs* that are subject to constant debate in the professional arena. Many clinicians and practitioners have questioned whether it is ethically right to circulate such material to parents and carers who, understandably, are left with the view that ADHD is a definite, proven medical disorder around which there is no controversy, and whose 'treatment' is similarly uncontroversial. Their decisions regarding the care of their children are based on such advice.

Why is there a false certainty?

This is a very difficult question to answer. It is important to acknowledge that 'false certainties' are not new in health – certainly not in mental health – any more than they are in other areas of life. Part of the reason for this is that people generally prefer issues to be clear-cut. On the whole, human beings do not cope well with uncertainty. Although this is a feature of our everyday life, it is perhaps most prevalent in the health field, where we expect there to be definitive answers rather than ideas, debates and theories. So far as children's mental health is concerned, there are significant differences in thinking and practice. In many ways it is unsurprising that the range of professional opinion and practice should be reflected in disagreements about attentional problems in children. What has been surprising is the rate at which ADHD as a diagnostic category has 'taken off', the rush to emphasise its biological credentials and legitimacy as a clinical construct, and the concurrent attempt to de-emphasise dissent and foster consensus.

International lack of consensus

This is exemplified by the publication of the International Consensus Statement in 2002 by a well-known supporter of ADHD, Russell Barkley, and his colleagues.[19] This paper was signed by a 'consortium of international scientists' claiming concern about 'inaccurate stories rendering ADHD a myth.' The paper seeks to present a united position on ADHD as a recognised medical disorder, and criticises the views of those who do not agree as 'wholly unscientific.' Critical literature is described as 'propaganda' and dissenters as 'fringe doctors' with a 'political agenda.' This Consensus Statement has been criticised by a number of practitioners and academics in the field, among them Joanna Moncrieff, Senior Lecturer in Social and Community Psychiatry at University College, London. In her paper entitled *'Is Psychiatry for Sale?'* she describes the statement by Barkley and his colleagues as 'an explicit attempt to cut short debate on these issues.'[20] Furthermore, Moncrieff has suggested that the authors should be obliged to declare their financial interests in this matter. Despite the view that Barkley and his colleagues are trying to promote, the title of the publication remains ironic – the reality is that there is anything but a consensus on ADHD. As psychiatrist Sami Timimi has pointed out, if there really were a proper consensus on ADHD, such a 'consensus' document would not be needed.[21]

Others have participated in the development and promotion of the 'false certainty', and their influence has been powerful, pervasive and purposeful. These are the pharmaceutical companies who make the drugs that are used to 'treat' ADHD. These will be discussed in the next two chapters.

CHAPTER 2

The psychopharmacology of ADHD

. . . and the drugs don't work, they just make things worse . . .
The Verve, *Urban Hymns*

Over the years, a number of different drugs have been used to treat hyperactivity. The use of stimulants to treat children labelled 'hyperactive' dates back as far as the 1930s, when an amphetamine, Benzedrine, was noted to have an impact on children's behaviour. In the late 1940s, another amphetamine, Dexedrine, was introduced, promising the same effect but at a lower dose. Soon after this, in 1954, a new drug, methylphenidate hydrochloride (MPH), was released. Although Dexedrine is still prescribed for ADHD, along with the 'combination' amphetamine, Adderall, by far the most frequently used stimulant is methylphenidate, which is taken, under one name or another, by 80–90% of children with a diagnosis of ADHD.

MPH is an amphetamine-like stimulant that acts on the central nervous system (CNS). It was first used to treat children with a diagnosis of hyperactivity in the 1960s, and is now most commonly used to treat ADHD in children and adults. Currently there are three main drugs on the market that contain MPH. These have the 'brand names' *Ritalin, Concerta* and *Equasym.* A methylphenidate 'patch' is awaiting approval.

How does MPH work?

Methylphenidate is a CNS stimulant that has similar properties to cocaine. Despite being a stimulant, it produces, among other things, a narrowing of attention. In the past, this was described as a 'paradoxical' effect (i.e. opposite to that expected) that occurred only in children with attention or hyperactivity 'disorders.' We now know that this is not the case. Like other forms of 'speed', MPH produces the same effect in everyone who takes it, whether they have a diagnosable disorder or not.

MPH is believed to work by acting on the dopamine receptors of the brain. However, we do not know exactly how, or why, it has the effect that it does. Believe it or not, *over half a century after it was first patented, we still do not really know how this drug affects the brain.*

Who takes Ritalin?

Most estimates suggest that more than 75% of methylphenidate prescriptions are written for children, with boys being about four times more likely than girls to be prescribed the drug.[1] Stimulant medication has been actively promoted by the drug companies as the treatment of choice for ADHD, and there have been huge increases in the numbers of prescriptions for the drug in recent years. There has been an increase in the number of Ritalin prescriptions in England between 1991, when only 2,000 were issued, and 2005, when a total of 359,100 prescriptions were issued. *This represents an 180-fold increase in Ritalin prescribing.*[2]

TABLE 2.1 Methylphenidate hydrochloride (Ritalin) prescriptions in England during the period 1991–2005

Year	Number of prescriptions
1991	2,000
1992	3,000
1993	4,000
1994	6,000
1997	92,000
1998	127,000
1999	158,000
2000	186,000
2001	208,000
2002	254,000[3]
2005	359,100[4]

The same data are presented as a graph in Figure 2.1.

These figures show enormous leaps in the prescribing of Ritalin. For example, in just one year, between 1996 and 1997, the UK jumped up from 30th place in the international league table of Ritalin prescribers to 9th place.[5] Critics in the UK fear that the rising trend in Ritalin prescribing is following that in the USA, where infants as young as 15 months have been prescribed the drug.[6]

Although the use of stimulants in the UK increased dramatically during the 1990s, only a fraction of children and adults in the UK take Ritalin compared with those in the USA (about 10%). Although it is a comparatively small consumer, the UK has nevertheless been identified by the United Nations International Narcotics Control Board as being among those countries that show a troubling increase in prescribing of stimulant drugs for children.[7]

Curiously, this leap in prescribing has come about at a time when we are told that mental health problems in children have remained fairly stable. In 2004, for instance, the findings of a survey conducted by the Office for National Statistics, on behalf of the Department of Health and the Scottish Executive, were published. The title of this report is *Mental Health of Children and Young People in Great Britain, 2004.*[8]

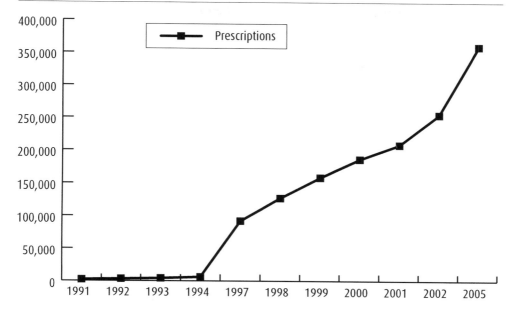

FIGURE 2.1 Ritalin prescriptions in England: 1991–2005.

The report begins by describing the prevalence of mental health disorders among 5- to 16-year-olds, and states that 'as a whole' there were no changes between 1999 and 2004 in the prevalence of conduct or hyperkinetic disorders among children aged 5–15 years. The report cites other European studies whose findings support this 'no change' position. However, if the prevalence has remained as stable as these studies suggest, why is it that Ritalin prescriptions have rocketed to the extent that they have? These figures suggest that the change was not in the incidence of 'ADHD'-type problems but in their *treatment*.

Rising concerns

Many mental health professionals, as well as parents, are concerned about the rate of increase in Ritalin prescriptions in the UK. As the figures confirm, there is indeed something to be concerned about. In December 2004, the BBC announced that there had been a 10-fold increase over 7 years in Scotland, prompting the NHS Quality Improvement Scotland (QIS) body to agree to audit the treatment of children with ADHD.[9]

Use of stimulants in different countries

The highest Ritalin consumer of all is the USA, which prescribes more Ritalin than all the other countries of the world combined. North America accounts for about 96% of the world's Ritalin consumption. The massive increase in the use of this drug has become a cause for concern worldwide. In fact, so many children are now taking the drug that the United Nations has called for an investigation by the World Health Organization.

Prescribing rates around the world vary enormously. Australia has increased its Ritalin consumption fairly rapidly in recent years, as has Spain. A comparative study published by Australian researchers in 2002 suggested that among the 10 countries they examined in North America, Australasia and Europe, there had been a 12% average total annual increase in consumption of psychostimulants in the 6 years from 1994 to 2000.[10] The study confirmed the 'big three' users as the USA, Canada and Australia.

In contrast, France, Denmark and Sweden continue to have low rates of Ritalin consumption. France has a population approaching 31 million people, who consumed just 100,000 Ritalin pills in 1998. Compare this with the *56.5 million pills* taken by Canadians, a population of almost equivalent size. Could it be that French and Canadian children are so very different? Most of us would guess not. What the figures reflect are probably the differences in how children and their problems are viewed in these two countries. For example, it has been suggested that French culture makes it more likely for children to be living in intact families. Perhaps even more importantly, child development has not yet been medicalised as it has in many other countries: in France, childhood is still viewed through the psycho–social 'lens'.*

Ritalin abuse

In the UK, methylphenidate is classified as a Class B medication. This means that it is a 'Controlled Drug' or 'CD.' As a class B drug, MPH is prescribed on a 'named person' basis only, which means that the prescription has to be handwritten. In addition, due to its status as a CD, MPH is kept in the pharmacy under strict conditions under lock and key. In the USA, MPH is classed as a Schedule II narcotic. This is the designation used for substances that have a recognised medical value but also a high potential for abuse. In Australia, it is classified as a Schedule 8 drug, which puts it in the same class as heroin.

Many parents whose children have been prescribed Ritalin are unaware that they are giving their children 'speed', and are even more surprised to learn of the growing 'black market' for Ritalin. The problem of Ritalin abuse has become widespread as prescription rates have risen and the drug has become more easily accessible in homes, schools, colleges and universities. In its 1994 report, the University of Michigan suggested that more high–school seniors in the USA were taking Ritalin illegally than were legally prescribed the drug. In 1996, the Drug Enforcement Agency reported that 30–50% of adolescents in drug treatment centres reported 'non–medical use' of Ritalin.†

---

* Further information can be found at the website for Stimulants Are Not The Answer (SANTA); www.santa.inuk. com/cerebrum.htm

† Data from the University of Michigan report, *Monitoring the Future*, cited in a press release by the Drug Enforcement Agency, October 1995.

How can a prescription drug that we are assured is safe to give to children be such an unknown quantity and have such a dangerous potential for misuse?

The answer lies partly in the way that Ritalin is used. Taken orally, MPH is slow-acting. This means that it is discharged into the system slowly, over a period of time. However, if the tablets are crushed and then snorted, it becomes fast-acting, producing a 'high' similar to that of cocaine or amphetamine (more rarely, it can be ground up, mixed with water, 'cooked' and injected intravenously). As a result, Ritalin misuse has become a growing trend in every country that prescribes it. Its similarities to cocaine have earned Ritalin the title 'kiddie cocaine.'

BOX 2.1 Ritalin – a 'soft' stimulant?

A study in 1995 by the research psychiatrist, Nora Volkow, confirmed the similarities between Ritalin and cocaine in their action on the brain and central nervous system.[11] Volkow and her colleagues found that the action of these drugs was identical. The only difference was the time that it took for Ritalin to leave the body. A more recent study by Volkow confirms these similarities but goes even further, reporting that Ritalin's effect on the dopamine system of the brain is even more potent that that of cocaine.[12]

Some researchers have found that Ritalin users are more likely than non-users to become cocaine users. They suggest that Ritalin, like amphetamine, changes the chemistry of the brain in such a way that it 'primes' it for cocaine. The cocaine has a stronger effect than it would have without this priming effect, amplifying the addiction risk.[13] Other studies have suggested that Ritalin use leads to higher rates of drug and alcohol use in adulthood.[*] They found that the effects were far-reaching, with evidence of higher rates of divorce, lower self-esteem and depression. Researchers found that more than 30% of the young Ritalin users they followed up dropped out of education, and 10% attempted suicide.

BOX 2.2 Kurt Cobain

According to his biographer, Charles Cross, Nirvana's Kurt Cobain believed that his use of Ritalin as a child led to his later abuse of other substances. He was prescribed Ritalin at the age of 7 years. His widow, Courtney Love, also took Ritalin as a child and is quoted by Cross as saying, 'When you're a kid and you get this drug that makes you feel that feeling, where else are you going to turn when you're an adult?'[14] Kurt Cobain committed suicide in 1994. He was 27 years old.

Others, too, have implicated Ritalin in their use of other drugs. The writer Elizabeth Wurtzel, author of *Prozac Nation*, documents her own Ritalin addiction in her book, *More, Now, Again*.[15] Her addiction began with a prescription from her psychiatrist.

---

* Brookhaven Laboratory researchers have been following up 5,000 children into adulthood, and have found that ADHD children treated with Ritalin exhibit higher rates of alcohol and drug use and are involved in more criminal activities and accidents compared with non-users.

She soon discovered another way to take her medication:

> I enjoy snorting up the Ritalin so much that after a couple of days I figure – what the hell? – I'll just take all of it that way . . . The only problem is that it hits very hard when I sniff it up, it goes right to my brain, so there's no chance for it to absorb into my bloodstream gradually . . . I try to maintain at least two hours between lines. I try.
>
> Then after a few days, I give up on trying . . . There are 6-year-olds who are given Ritalin for attention deficit hyperactivity disorder (ADHD), and some of them take more than a hundred milligrams a day. If a kid in the first grade can handle it, why shouldn't I be able to?

Elizabeth Wurtzel was not alone in asking herself this question.

Such was the level of concern about Ritalin that the US Drug Enforcement Administration (DEA) posted the following information on its website in 1995 – *more than a decade ago.*

NEWS RELEASE

FOR IMMEDIATE RELEASE
20 October 1995

Methylphenidate
- Methylphenidate (MPH), most commonly known as Ritalin, ranks in the top 10 most frequently reported controlled pharmaceuticals stolen from licensed handlers.
- Abuse of MPH can lead to marked tolerance and severe psychic dependence.
- Organized drug-trafficking groups in a number of states have utilized various schemes to obtain MPH for resale on the illicit market.
- MPH is abused by diverse segments of the population, from health care professions and children to street addicts.
- A significant number of children and adolescents are diverting or abusing MPH medication intended for the treatment of ADHD.
- In 1994, a national high-school survey (Monitoring the Future) indicated that more seniors in the US abuse Ritalin than are prescribed Ritalin legitimately.
- Students are giving and selling their medication to classmates, who are crushing and snorting the powder like cocaine. In March 1995, two deaths in Mississippi and Virginia were associated with this activity.
- DAWN (Drug Abuse Warning Network) statistics on estimated emergency-room mentions indicate that there were 271 mentions in 1990, 657 mentions in 1991, 1044 mentions in 1992, and 725 in 1993 (of which 28% to 40% were associated with abuse for dependence or psychological effects). The number of mentions for MPH was significantly greater than mentions for Schedule III stimulants (6 mentions in 1992 and 1 mention in 1993 for all Schedule III stimulants).
- The US manufactures and consumes five times more MPH than the rest of the world combined.

- MPH aggregate production quota has increased almost sixfold since 1990.
- Every indicator available, including scientific abuse liability studies, actual abuse, paucity of scientific studies on possible adverse effects associated with long-term use of stimulants, divergent prescribing practices of US physicians, and lack of concurrent medical treatment and follow-up, urges greater caution and more restrictive use of MPH.

(Drug Enforcement Administration, 1995)
For original, go to: www.dea.gov/pubs/pressrel/pr951020.htm

Side-effects of ADHD drugs

Of course, there are side-effects associated with the use of any drug. Now that the Internet is the communication vehicle of choice in hospitals, clinics and other health-care settings, health warnings and notices of the immediate withdrawal or suspension of particular drugs appear in practitioners' 'Inboxes' on an alarmingly regular basis. They really bring home the experimental nature of much drug treatment. Drugs that have been thought to be safe and prescribed freely for years are suddenly withdrawn due to serious side-effects and even deaths associated with their use. Members of the general public rarely get to hear of these developments.

Hyperactivity drugs are no exception. For example, *Adderall XR*, the combination amphetamine produced by Shire Pharmaceuticals, was suspended in February 2005 in Canada because of safety concerns. These included sudden deaths, heart-related deaths, and strokes in children and adults taking usual recommended doses of Adderall and Adderall XR. Health Canada, the Canadian drug regulatory agency, reported that the deaths were not associated with overuse, misuse or abuse. A total of 14 deaths occurred in children and 6 deaths in adults. The ban was reversed 6 months later, not because the drug was found to be safe, but because there was not enough evidence to prove that it increased the risk of heart-related deaths.

Atomoxetine

In the USA, atomoxetine (trade name *Strattera*) was hailed as the first non-stimulant drug to be approved by the Food and Drug Administration for the treatment of ADHD. Not only was it a non-controlled substance, but also it was approved for use in both adults and children. Strattera is manufactured by Eli Lilly.

One of the main differences between atomoxetine and drugs like methylphenidate or amphetamine is that atomoxetine acts to make more of the hormone *norepinephrine* available in the brain. Thus it was heralded as a great step forward: no more amphetamines – this was much safer. Not so, argued the critics. Just because this adrenalin-like hormone is a substance that is naturally produced in the body, that doesn't mean it is safe to increase its availability (after all, too much insulin would kill you). Where is the evidence that effectively raising levels of norepinephrine is any safer than introducing a synthetic stimulant into the nervous systems of children? According to the psychiatrist Grace Jackson, it is a matter of semantics. Atomoxetine meets all three of the World Health Organization's criteria for psychostimulants – it is chemically derived from a stimulant, its pharmacological effects are the same, and it has the same behavioural effects.[16] Critics argued that *no* drugs which affect the functioning of the brain and central nervous system should be considered safe. This argument proved to be prophetic. Predictably, after trumpeting atomoxetine as the 'safer' alternative to Ritalin, worrying side-effects began to be reported.

In 2004, Lilly added a health warning to the Stattera label. They warned users to stop their medication if they developed jaundice or liver problems. *This was after two million people had been taking the drug.* In March 2005, Lilly added a further warning about possible suicidal thoughts. As if this isn't worrying enough in itself, we have to remember that the wheels of the information machine turn very slowly, even now in the age of the Internet (and in some countries they may not turn at all). It took a good two months for the warning about potential liver disorders to reach clinical staff in the UK, and a whole six months for staff to be circulated with information warning them of the risk of 'suicidal thoughts/ behaviour' in atomoxetine users.*

What about Ritalin?

Dexedrine, Adderall and Strattera all have side-effects, but this chapter is focusing primarily on Ritalin because the vast majority of children with an ADHD diagnosis are taking this drug.

So far, the known potential side–effects of Ritalin are as follows.

Short-term effects

These include the following symptoms:

- reduced physical growth
- headaches
- abdominal pain, loss of appetite, upset stomach, nausea or vomiting
- sleep difficulties
- palpitations, changes in heart rate and blood pressure
- jitteriness, nervousness or irritability
- lethargy, dizziness or drowsiness
- social withdrawal and suicidal tendencies
- skin rashes and itching.

Long-term effects

High doses of Ritalin over a longer period produce the following symptoms:

- loss of appetite
- tremors and muscle twitching
- fevers, headaches and convulsions
- irregular heartbeat and respiration

---

* Clinical staff working for the NHS obtain regular bulletins from the Department of Health in the form of public health link broadcasts. The public health link warning of potential hepatic disorders was issued on 3 February 2005, and the one alerting staff to potential suicidal thoughts was issued on 29 September 2005.

- anxiety and restlessness
- paranoia, hallucinations and delusions
- excessive repetitive movements
- formication (sensation of insects or worms crawling under the skin).[*]

Research has identified that methylphenidate might cause chromosomal damage linked to cancer.[†]

Deaths from Ritalin

Some children have died as a direct result of taking Ritalin. These children died not because they were taking the drug illegally or because they overdosed on it. They died while they were taking the prescribed dose, following their ADHD diagnosis. Among these children were Shania Dunkle (aged 10 years), Matthew Smith (aged 14), Stephanie Hall (aged 11) and Randy Steele (aged 9). You can read about all of these children on the Internet. Matthew Smith's father has posted details of his son's death, officially recorded as 'death caused from long-term use of methylphenidate (Ritalin)', and you can read about Matthew at www.ritalindeath.com.

According to the child neurologist and ADHD critic Dr Fred Baughman, 2,993 adverse reactions to Ritalin were recorded between 1990 and 1997. Of these, there were 160 deaths and 569 hospitalisations, 126 of which involved cardiovascular adverse reactions.[17] Since this, the numbers of deaths have continued to rise – with 26 more children dying by 2000.[18] How many have died since then is not clear.

Long-term effects on the brain

Side-effects – and deaths – aside, many child specialists are worried about the potential long-term effects of MPH, as well as other psychoactive medications, on the still-developing brains of children. This is because when we use medications such as these, we are effectively engaging in an experiment. Let's consider the brain for a few minutes and the way in which drugs exert an effect in the first place.

The blood–brain barrier

The first challenge for any drug is to pass through the *blood–brain barrier*. This is a very important mechanism that prevents harmful substances from passing through the blood into the tissues of the brain. It is the means by which the brain protects itself. When new medications are developed, scientists have to find ways of getting around this protective mechanism by molecular manipulation. Once they have done this, they then have to navigate their way around the most complex organ of the body.

---

[*] *Source:* Bailey WJ. Indiana Prevention Resource Center (IPRC) Factline.

[†] Research reported in February 2005 and conducted at the Anderson Cancer Centre was cited on Newswise, 24 February 2005 (see References).

Complexity of the brain

The brain is incredibly complex, consisting of over 100 billion neurons, each of which makes thousands and thousands of connections with other cells via substances called neurotransmitters. Other kinds of cells, called glia, are even more numerous. In fact, there are so many cells in the brain that it is difficult to find a word to describe their number. Psychoactive medications affect all of these cells and all of the processes in which they are engaged. Attempts to target specific sites of the brain result in the 'ripple effect',* which means that the effects can be far-reaching and unpredictable.

How Ritalin is believed to act on the brain

As discussed earlier, Ritalin is assumed to act on the brain by increasing the amount of dopamine available. MPH is a dopamine *reuptake inhibitor*, which means that it increases the level of the dopamine neurotransmitter in the brain. It does this by partially blocking the transporters that would ordinarily remove dopamine from the synapses (the communication 'spaces' between receptors, across which messages are sent and received).

As the brain is so very complex, the action of a psychoactive medication is anything but straightforward or predictable. First, the claim that a particular medication can act on a single target site, like a miniature 'guided missile', without affecting other cells and other systems in the brain has been dismissed by a number of authors. Many of these are well-known psychiatrists, such as Grace Jackson and Peter Breggin, who have devoted much of their careers to alerting readers in Europe and North America to the dangers of psychoactive drugs. The brain is not only complex but also extremely adaptable, and therefore reacts to protect itself from these toxic substances that would ordinarily not get past the blood–brain barrier. It responds in such ways as developing more receptors when it detects a need to – hence more 'side-effects' and other unforeseen negative consequences of the 'ripple effect.'*

It seems incredible, then, that drug companies should see fit to release information, promotional material and advertisements which suggest that the brain is as simple as the diagram you probably drew in your exercise book at school. In this simplified brain, targeting a specific site becomes an easy process. The 'cause' of whatever mental health problem is being described is a safe and simple neurobiological certainty – something that can be fixed as easily as a battery in need of recharging.

The reality is that we already know from nearly two decades of studies on antipsychotic medications that these medications have very severe long-term side-effects – the magic, inter-neuronal 'guided missile' is a myth. Unfortunately, it is a myth that continues to be pedalled.

Why does this matter? Because the information we are given is critical to the decisions that we make. In order to make choices about treatment – whatever that treatment may be – we need to have all of the available information in order to weigh

---

* This is an expression used by Grace Jackson to describe the wider effects of supposedly safe, targeted psychiatric drugs. In: Jackson G. *Rethinking Psychiatric Drugs: a guide for informed consent.* Bloomington, IN: AuthorHouse; 2005.

up the pros and cons. This is the basis of *informed consent*. Unfortunately, it seems that we are unlikely to be as informed about drug treatment as we should be. As parents, if we don't know what the side-effects or long-term effects are, how can we make a properly informed choice? As for children, do they even get a choice?

When is a toddler not a toddler . . .?

Despite the many concerns that have already been raised, and although it is clearly not recommended for children under 6 years of age, Ritalin is being prescribed to an increasing number of children below this age. In the USA and Canada a worrying trend seems to be developing whereby children are being medicated earlier and earlier. In 2000, it was reported that there had been a threefold increase in the prescribing of psychoactive medications to pre-school children over a 5-year period.[19] In general, it seems that between 3% and 4% of pre-school children, some as young as 15 months, are being prescribed psychostimulant medication.[20]

It is difficult to access the kind of information that would indicate some kind of trend in the UK. However, my own clinical experience and that of my colleagues working in child and adolescent mental health clinics in the Midlands suggest a rising number of referrals of under-fives *specifically for an ADHD diagnosis*. My own clinic referrals included one 4-year-old who 'cannot have a proper conversation', pre-school children who 'can't pay attention', and others who 'can't sit still' and are 'wilful.' If, like me, your first thoughts are that these sound like descriptions of ordinary pre-schoolers, you probably have children of your own. You would also be quite right.

In my experience there has been a startling increase in the number of referrals to mental health agencies of children whose behaviour is entirely within the normal range for a pre-school child. Even more worrying has been my experience of referrals of very young children who are already known to be on the Child Protection Register and already understood to have a home environment that is emotionally impoverished, traumatic or otherwise lacking in nurturance. For this group of children it is particularly worrying that it is *their* behaviour that is singled out as requiring 'treatment.' Presumably the child is in need of 'fixing', whereas the family can remain unaltered.

To me, such referrals represent something of a sea change in attitude. Whereas previously the pre-school focus was on social support and education, it now seems to be much more medical. The consequences include an apparent deskilling of many excellent and otherwise sensible social care and child development practitioners who are also caught up in this pseudoscientific story of ADHD and how it should be treated.

Why do we continue to have such faith in prescription drugs?

On the basis of the information reviewed so far, you might be forgiven for wondering why on earth we continue – blindly, it seems – to put our faith in these drugs. There may be several reasons, some of which are listed below.

- We are told they are safe.
- We are told they are tested.
- They are regulated.
- We have respect for high-status professionals, such as doctors. As we all know, 'doctor knows best.'
- Our faith in prescription drugs has been carefully cultivated over decades by pharmaceutical companies who have promoted a view of mental health problems as medical illnesses that can be 'cured' by drugs. Our thinking about ADHD is entirely in keeping with this view.

Mixed messages: drugs are bad – except when they're good

In general, our acquiescence in this process has been quite astonishing given the increasing levels of concern about pollutants, food additives and colourings, genetically modified ingredients and other 'unnatural' substances. Apparently these concerns do not extend to the drugging of our children. Similarly, industrialised societies all over the world are made increasingly aware of the adverse effects of tobacco, alcohol and drugs. Most parents would not dream of giving non-prescription drugs or alcohol to their children. And if they did, they would very quickly find themselves the subject of a Social Services investigation.

Yet thousands of us every day give our children drugs whose side-effects are *already* known to be serious and whose long-term effects on the developing brain remain an unknown entity.

Gore Vidal echoes the thoughts of many when he criticises this kind of double-think. 'Although drugs are "immoral" and must be kept from the young', he surmises, 'thousands of schools pressure parents to give the drug Ritalin to any child who may, sensibly, show any sign of boredom in the classroom. Ritalin renders the child docile if not comatose. Side-effects? Stunted growth, facial tics, agitation and aggression, insomnia, appetite loss, headaches, stomach pains and seizures. Marijuana would be far less harmful.'[21]

But who would give their child an after-breakfast spliff or a pre-class shot of alcohol just because it 'works'? After all, lots of things 'work' (whatever that means), but that doesn't necessarily make them right. As my friend Jo said to me recently, 'Beating the hell out of someone might have the desired effect sometimes, but that wouldn't make it right.' Do we really think it's all right to give our children drugs because they seem to calm them down?

A dangerous journey

Given that so many negative effects of medications have come to the fore only after longer-term use, we should be worried about young children who have already embarked on a long-term drug journey with Ritalin. Many children who are referred to local children's mental health practitioners have been taking this drug for years. In my own experience, it is not unusual to meet children who have been taking it for as long as 7 or 8 years (some even longer), often without the requisite monitoring and without any real observable benefits. To give the drug companies their due, this is not what they would recommend. Their literature advises that careful monitoring is essential and that if the drug does not seem to be having any benefit it should be discontinued after 1 month.

The drug companies also recommend 'drug holidays' for children taking Ritalin. These are drug-free periods during which time the child's behaviour can be observed. However, it is not uncommon to see children who have never had a 'drug holiday', despite being long-term users of Ritalin. This is the reality of drug use in everyday life – it is always different to what manufacturers suggest it is.

There are many reasons why these children continue on their medications in the way they do. Often they are children whose family circumstances are insecure or chaotic, which means that they move around a lot or have frequent changes of carer, and often of doctors as well. Many of these children are looked after by the local authority in children's homes or in foster care. This can mean that prescriptions just continue to get repeated, once the child or young person has been given the label 'ADHD.' Social workers frequently refer to mental health teams because one of the newly admitted children in a children's home has a diagnosis of ADHD and they need to find someone to continue to prescribe the medication.

The philosophy in my clinical team was never to do this, but to suggest instead that such a request provides a good opportunity to reassess the child. Some would-be referrers have not liked this response, and have simply found someone else to do the prescribing. In cases where they have taken the opportunity for a reassessment I have not found a single case where the original diagnosis has been borne out. (There will be more on misdiagnosis in Chapter 7.)

When the child doesn't change

Sometimes we don't have this opportunity to intervene. The medication is just continued because *the child doesn't change* – the ADHD is still believed to be exerting a strong influence on the child and their family, and it is felt that there is a need to continue or even, in my experience, to increase the medication. In cases where medication is being monitored adequately and the child has a 'drug holiday', this sometimes provides further proof that the child 'hasn't got better', as again *the problems for which the family originally sought help are often still there, and perhaps even worse.* (Of course they are – we haven't done anything about them.) Drug holidays serve to confirm this for them, and they become anxious that the drug is going to be withdrawn. In the mean time, children continue to take this drug at a time when, as we have already seen, their brains are still developing. Many feel that this is just too great a risk.

Grace Jackson, in her lectures on the limitations and unintended consequences of biological psychiatry, uses a witty but nevertheless chilling parallel. She cites the work of Isaac Newton, reminding us of his *third law of motion* – 'for every action there is an equal and opposite reaction.' Jackson's own variation of this, which she calls *Jackson's law of biopsychiatry*, runs thus:

For every action, there is an unequal and frequently unpredictable reaction.[22]

While in some cases we never know what to expect, some of these reactions are not so unpredictable. In 1998, Peter Breggin listed the negative short- and long-term effects of stimulant medication. They make sobering reading.

Negative short- and long-term effects of psychostimulants

1 Psychostimulants can cause irreversible brain damage and dysfunction. This is known with a high degree of scientific probability with regard to amphetamine and methamphetamine, and with a high level of suspicion with regard to MPH.
2 Psychostimulants cause multiple adverse effects, including a variety of cardiac and CNS effects, such as obsessive-compulsive disorder, depression and even mania. The CNS effects confuse doctors, leading inappropriately to further psychiatric diagnosis and medication rather than to drug withdrawal.
3 Psychostimulants impair growth, including that of the brain.
4 Psychostimulants work by suppressing spontaneity and sociability, by enforcing obsessive-compulsive perseverative behaviour, and by isolating the child from normal outside influences.
5 These drugs should not be used to treat children for behavioural, emotional or school problems.[23]

The fact is – and it is worth repeating – no one knows what effect Ritalin is having on the brains of our children, and we shall not know this for many years to come. If the drugs that deal with 'symptoms' also affect and possibly damage the still-developing brain, does the 'cure' come at too high a price?

The long-term effects of MPH on the brain are simply unknown. The brains of children are still developing, and some areas of the brain continue to develop until about the age of 30, notably the frontal lobes, which are vital to *executive functioning*, such as managing thoughts and feelings. Much concern has therefore been expressed about the possible detrimental effect of MPH over time, but no long-term studies have yet been undertaken.

The action of MPH on the brain and the way in which it is deemed to 'work' in children labelled as having ADHD is a post-hoc explanation. That is, it has developed *after experiments in mass medication*, in common with other psychoactive drugs. In other words, our children are continuing to act as a means of gathering this information. *They are the first wave of experimental subjects in the Ritalin Longitudinal (long-term) Study.*

And as for all the debate about whether or not these drugs 'work', the latest evidence suggests that they don't. On 20 September 2005, ABC News Online reported on a study conducted by the Drug Effectiveness Review Project at Oregon State University, which reviewed more than 2,000 studies.[24] The conclusion was that there is little evidence that the drugs which are used to treat ADHD actually work or are safe in the long term.

We have been prescribing this drug for children for decades now, without having the answers to some extremely important questions, and with scarce evidence that the drug really works. Notwithstanding all the risks involved, the effects of drug treatment appear to be highly questionable. Given what we know about the dangers of Ritalin, as well as the dangers of what we don't know, is it really worth the risk?

Isn't it time we stopped this mass experiment?

CHAPTER 3

The drug companies

We are living in times when we seek certainty, even in places where there is none. In the twenty-first century, at a time when we are riddled with anxieties about health and mortality, no area is more likely to be the subject of this search than health. As we search, we look to science to give us the answers – nowadays it is in science that we trust. But faith in science can serve many purposes, not least of which is the desire to affirm our beliefs that we are only partially responsible for what happens to us – if at all. Some other, larger power must be at work, controlling our destinies. This idea can be quite comforting, as we live with our many imperfections. It can also be helpful to us. As adults, we are good at seeking to absolve ourselves of responsibility for all sorts of things – the way we eat, drink, smoke, use drugs, gain weight, gamble, to list just a few. It works very well for us to look to 'genes' and biology to explain the way we are. It is so much more acceptable to blame our genes for some of our characteristics, rather than ourselves. How much better it feels to blame our children's difficulties on their genetic or physiological make-up, rather than on what we do to them. Our ever-increasing faith in the progress of science makes us look towards science to answer many of our questions. What we have read so far suggests that sometimes we might be looking in the wrong place.

We have already seen that there are a number of reasons why people trust their doctors and have faith in the medicines that they prescribe, but this is not conclusive. There is another reason why, as parents and clinicians, we are happy to go along with what is no more than a mass experiment in medication. This is because of the information we are given that seems to speak with such authority. Much of this tells us just the opposite of some of the information I have presented so far here. It suggests that giving our children stimulant medication is the right thing to do, that we need to do more of it and, furthermore, that if we *don't* do this we might be harming them.

To help us to understand why so many of us are medicating our children in such large numbers, we need to look at the information that parents and carers – and their doctors – are given, and how the 'prevailing view' on ADHD and what is best for children is developed and maintained. For this, we need to look at the drug companies.

Drugs and big business

The drug companies have a major influence over the information that reaches parents, teachers, medical practitioners and other clinical staff working in the field of children's health. As profit-making industries their primary interest is, of course, to sell as much of their product as possible – an understandable motive in the business world. However, the substantial part played by drug companies as providers of information and the special relationship that appears to have been cultivated with psychiatrists raise a number of questions, not least about the potential conflict of interest inherent in such a blurring of boundaries between private profit and public interest.

Over the course of the last 20–25 years, drugs have become big business. The pharmaceutical industry has undergone phenomenal development during this period, from a relatively small group of companies with specific areas of focus to its current position 'among the most profitable industries on earth.'[1] Not only is the drug business booming, it is also competitive and increasingly predatory, spending significant amounts of money on marketing and promotion to extend its spheres of influence. Some of the methods employed in the process have led to concerns that doctors, as well as the general public, are being deliberately misled. At the same time, there is growing criticism of the increasingly incestuous relationships between medical practice and the drug industry.

The big sell: marketing tactics used by the drug companies

Drug company marketing is extensive and includes the following methods:

- advertising and promotion
- 'hospitality' for medical practitioners
- consultancy
- funding for medical education, training and conferences
- funding for research
- dissemination of information
- news groups/Internet support groups
- 'ghost writing' of medical articles
- funding for pro-drug patient and carer groups, such as CHADD* in the USA and ADDISS† in the UK; these organisations also run Internet support groups
- political lobbying and direct funding of political bodies, including drug regulatory agencies.

Why is it that drug companies invest so much time, effort and money in these things? The answer is *because they work*. They work very well and the drug companies spend huge amounts of money on these kinds of activities because they know this. One drug company can easily spend more than a large multinational company, such as Pepsi or Budweiser, on advertising alone.‡

---

* CHADD is the acronym for Children and Adults with Attention Deficit Disorder.

† The acronym ADDISS stands for Attention Deficit Disorder Information and Support Service.

‡ In 2000, the drug company Vioxx spent 161 million dollars on advertising. This was more than Pepsi and Budweiser

Read through the list of their activities very quickly and they might seem fairly innocuous, but now read it again – slowly. Each one of these things plays an important part in shaping thinking about ADHD, each one vigorously promotes stimulant medication as the treatment of choice, and each one includes conduct that is highly contentious. Let us look each of these activities in turn.

Advertising and promotion

In Europe, drug companies are not allowed to advertise directly to the public, as they are in other countries, such as the USA, where data suggest that there is a direct relationship between the amount spent on consumer advertising and growth in sales. Instead, they have to rely on other, non-direct means of communication. They can of course advertise their products to doctors, and they do this via medical journals and promotional leaflets. They also have other, highly successful ways of getting their message across.

Drug companies routinely offer gifts and other inducements to doctors (visit your own GP and have a glance round the office). Many of these gifts will be in the form of 'branded' calendars, pens, Post-it notes, coffee mugs, desk clocks and the like. However, some can be more significant, involving the use of exclusive hotels, expensive dinners and even trips abroad disguised as promotional or educational activity.[2] 'No Free Lunch' is one of a growing number of campaigns that are encouraging medical doctors to reject the drug companies' marketing practices. Bob Goodman, founder of 'No Free Lunch', highlights the fact that even small, seemingly innocuous gifts can have far-reaching effects. He often draws an analogy between drug company incentives and buying a drink for someone else at a bar. This simple act gives rise to some expectation on behalf of the recipient, namely that the person will buy you one back.

Goodman suggests that drug company tactics have a similar effect, which he believes takes the form of prescriptions for patients.[*] Advertising research has been telling us for years that, when people are given a choice, they will choose the product they have already seen or heard of, rather than a completely new one. Drug company advertising is no different. Studies show that even small gifts influence doctors' prescribing decisions – even if they just receive a pen bearing the company's logo and the name of a particular drug, which almost all doctors do, they will be more likely to prescribe that drug.[3]

'Hospitality' for medical practitioners

Drug company representatives have been described as 'the stealth bombers of medicine',[4] so great is their impact on would-be prescribers. Readers who have any familiarity with hospital settings will probably have encountered 'the drug rep' who comes along with a free buffet lunch (and freebies) for lunchtime seminars – a fixture for doctors at most hospitals. Some healthcare readers may also be familiar with such

---

each spent, according to the National Institute for Health Care Management. Moncrieff J. *Is Psychiatry for Sale?* Maudsley Discussion Paper. London: Institute of Psychiatry; 2003.

[*] You can read more about 'No Free Lunch' (and even take the pledge) at www.nofreelunch.org

things as free breakfast symposia at conferences and conventions, at which booklets and information (and more freebies) will be disseminated. Some may even have been recipients of travel funds, and 'product demonstration' dinners. Others may recall 'sponsored' study days, where drug companies have paid for the venue and a nice lunch. Depending on the perceived importance of such events to the sponsoring company, what's on offer can range from the basic to the very grand. Dressed up as support for education and training events, such 'hospitality' merely provides further opportunities for advertising, promotion and extension of the drug companies' professional networks.

BOX 3.1 The hard sell

On 14 February 2006, *The Guardian* published a brief article headed 'Drug firm censured for lapdancing junket.' It described how the staff of 'one of the world's largest drug companies' treated doctors to trips to greyhound racing events and lapdancing venues, and gave them Wimbledon Centre Court tickets. The company, Abbott Laboratories, was reprimanded for breaching the code of the Association of the British Pharmaceutical Industry (ABPI), and was suspended from its board of management for a period of 6 months. Abbott Laboratories was reported in the same article as making £2 billion (US$3.4 billion) profit in the previous financial year on worldwide sales of over US$ 22 million.[5]

Despite attempts to curb the excesses of drug company promotional activities, these remain as much of a problem as ever (*see* Box 3.1). Des Spence, UK spokesperson for 'No Free Lunch', has commented:

> the amount of hospitality received by the medical profession compared to other public services is, in my opinion, a complete disgrace. If you had any other public servants, like civil servants or teachers or policemen, receiving that level of hospitality, there would be a public outcry. There is this idea that doctors are somehow different from other people . . . it is difficult for doctors to hear this. It is so ingrained in them that they do not want to see it as a problem.[6]

The House of Commons enquiry into the influence of the pharmaceutical industry led to an amusing exchange on the subject of how to influence your doctor (*see* Box 3.2).

The pharmaceutical industry employs about 83,000 people directly, one in ten of whom are drug representatives.[7] In March 2006, the Consumers' Union of the USA presented information on their website which suggested that there was one drug rep for every nine doctors. If you think this is a high ratio, perhaps you didn't listen to an earlier BBC Radio 4 programme, in which it was suggested that there was now in fact *one drug rep for every doctor*.[8] Clearly, the drug companies must think it's worth it. And it is. In 2003, Shire Pharmaceuticals recorded sales of the ADHD combination amphetamine Adderall XR of over US$ 115 million just in the first quarter of 2003. This represented growth of 86% compared with the previous year.[9] Earlier, a 1999 estimate suggested that Novartis generated an increase in its stock-market value of

US$ 1,236 for every child prescribed Ritalin. Based on this estimate, the company would have had an increased stock-market value of over US$ 10 million since 1991.[10] That's over US$ 1.3 million a year – just from this one drug.

BOX 3.2 Doctor, Doctor!

Q94: Can I ask a naive question? GPs are very busy people. We hear constantly that they have no time for more than 5 minutes per patient. Why are they wasting their time seeing pharmaceutical companies?

Dr Spence: It is not a naive question. The reason is that you know these people. I feel slightly awkward about being here because I do not want to seem unkind to the people I have known for years and years, but I feel like I have to be. The reason we see them is because you have a personal contact with them. Often, certainly, in the areas that I work in, they provide lunch on a daily basis to many of the doctors and nurses in the area.

Q: So when I want an early appointment with my GP, I'm going about it the wrong way. I should offer to take him out to dinner.[11]

Consultancy

Another way in which drug companies can extend their influence is by linking with prescribers through paid consultancy work. Consultancy fees can be as high as £5,000 for an hour-long lecture. In reality, many of these arrangements represent little more than 'loyalty payments' to doctors for simply continuing to prescribe the company's drugs. Unfortunately, at the time of writing, it is difficult to keep track of such payments, as registers of financial dealing are not kept by hospital or general practitioners.

Tactics like this raise important questions about the appropriateness of companies seeking to influence doctors' decision making and prescribing. After all, if your doctor is being paid to prescribe a certain drug for you, how can you be sure that this won't influence the next decision he makes about which drug you need? This question arose during investigations in 2004 into Schering-Plough, one of the world's biggest drug companies. Gardiner Harris of the *New York Times*, reporting on these investigations, wrote:

> At the heart of the various investigations into drug industry marketing is the question of whether drug companies are persuading doctors – often through payoffs – to prescribe drugs that patients do not need or should not use.[12]

Funding for medical education, training and conferences

This, too, is an area that has mushroomed in size in recent years. Joseph Ross and colleagues in the USA, reviewing providers and sponsors of medical education, commented on the 'tremendous size and recent growth' of medical education services suppliers, as well as the dominance of the pharmaceutical industry in these services. They summarise many people's concerns in their comment that 'to permit for-profit companies to provide physician education is to sanction a clear conflict of interest.'[13] The conflict, of course, lies in the content of such education and how information is framed – in other words, right at its heart.

In the UK, the House of Commons Health Committee heard in 2005 that more than half of further education training for doctors is now funded by the drug industry. And it is not only doctors who are being trained by the drug companies. In 2003, GlaxoSmithKline funded diplomas in respiratory disease and diabetes management for 434 nurses. We can expect nurses to be increasingly targeted by the industry, as many of them have now been trained to prescribe medication (over 25,500 in the UK during 2004). They are part of a rising number of 'non-medical prescribers' that looks set to include pharmacists next, before extending the prescribing network still further.

It has been suggested that drug company sponsorship of education and training can lead to incorrect diagnoses as a result of focusing too heavily during training on diseases that can be treated by expensive new drugs. Peter Davies, consultant respiratory physician at the Cardiothoracic Centre and University Hospital Aintree in Liverpool, is only one of a number of doctors who argue that the balance of training is being adversely affected by such funding.[14]

In 2003, the Accreditation Council for Continuing Medical Education (CME) tried through its guidelines to ban drug company involvement in CME. This provoked outrage among drug companies and led to less stringent demands for regulation of their activities, rather than an outright ban. In April 2004, the first global standards for CME were developed by medical education accreditors from the USA and Europe. Core issues were responsibility for content, funding that is unrestricted (i.e. not contingent on any particular view being adopted), and disclosure of financial arrangements and potential conflicts of interest. The cynics among you might already be thinking that the fact that these are 'guidelines' means that they can be 'creatively' circumvented by those who really wish to do so. And, indeed, continuing education for doctors seems to have proceeded exactly as before. The consensus has been described by one of those involved as 'an acceptable compromise', by which I'm guessing he means acceptable to the drug companies and a compromise of everyone else's principles. Although the Accreditation Council has stated that the commercial interests of those providing education 'must be resolved', it neglects to tell us what will happen if they are not.[15]

Funding for research

It has been suggested that over 70% of research into drug treatment is funded by the drug companies themselves.[16] While not necessarily invalidating the research in question, such funding surely raises an important question about conflict of interest. Critics of drug-company-sponsored research point out that whoever pays for the research is crucial. The paymaster, they suggest, determines not only how the research is conducted, but also what gets reported (and what does not) once the study is completed. The resulting piece of research is likely to have been significantly affected by its funding source, but readers will be unaware of this, as well as what might have been deliberately left out.

One such example is the National Institute for Mental Health (NIMH) Multi-modal Treatment Study for ADHD (known as the MTA study). This is the study that proved to be so influential in making stimulant medication the treatment of choice for ADHD. The MTA study has been widely criticised, not least for its methodological flaws. However, many feel that it is not its methodology that invalidates it, but its drug company sponsorship and associations. (A critique of the MTA study is summarised in Appendix 1.)

It is quite remarkable that researchers and practitioners do not seem to accept this as a problem. One of the MTA study researchers was Dr Russell Barkley, an influential figure in the ADHD world, and considered to be a leading expert on ADHD. Barkley admits to taking money from drug companies for consultancy and 'speaking engagements.' However, he does not see this as problematic because it represents only 'a small proportion' of his income. Like many other doctors and academic psychiatrists, he seems to think he is immune to such influences. However, research suggests that he is wrong.

Given the inevitable interest in the outcomes of research, as well as in publicising it, it is difficult to imagine how drug company funding can be perceived as being in any way neutral. Nevertheless, it continues to be a widespread practice.

One widely-cited example is that of the *New England Journal of Medicine*, which in 2000 published a paper on the antidepressant nefazadone, but *did not have sufficient space* to print all of the financial interests of its authors. It also struggled to identify an academic psychiatrist who could write an editorial on the subject. The problem was not one of finding a suitable psychiatrist, but of finding one who did not also have concurrent financial ties with companies that make antidepressants.[17]

Drug companies therefore have a massive influence on what gets published. As a result, they play a key role in shaping views among healthcare practitioners and the public on health – and mental health – issues. Yet their influence goes still further, as they have the power to ensure that negative studies remain unpublished, block publication, or even change the content of papers.[18]

BOX 3.3 Dirty tricks

Dr P Wilmshurst:

One reason I am here is that I was offered a bribe of two years' salary not to publish research which was counter to the interests of the company making the drug. I know other people were influenced because of that not to publish – not because of bribes but pressure was put on researchers working on the same drug.[19]

(Evidence of Dr P Wilmshurst to the House of Commons Health Committee on the influence of the pharmaceutical industry)

It is often the case that research data are very selectively reported, and there are many ways in which drug companies do this, from deliberately withholding unfavourable reports to making sure that the research methodology is likely to produce results that are in their favour. Sometimes procedures themselves hide negative outcomes. For example, in trials of antidepressants known as selective serotonin reuptake inhibitors (SSRIs), the research data were coded in a way that masked serious problems with the drugs. Suicidal people were coded under the heading 'nausea' or 'treatment unresponsiveness', and children who became suicidal were coded as 'emotionally labile.' Children who became aggressive or even homicidal were coded as 'hostile.'[20]

BOX 3.4 More dirty tricks

Dr Wilmshurst again:

> When I published a paper on the side-effects of the drug [amrinone] in the *BMJ*, I was contacted by a regulator in the Netherlands Committee for the Evaluation of Medicines, who pointed out that he did not understand our paper because on our clinical record cards the side-effects were not reported. I had a copy of my clinical record cards and the documents he had were a forgery from the drug company. The company had altered our clinical record cards and the documents he had were a forgery from the company. The company had altered our clinical record cards, omitting side-effects.[21]

On hearing some of the tactics used by the drug companies, Sir Richard Sykes, Rector of Imperial College, London, remarked to the House of Commons Health Committee, 'Obviously, like anything else in the world today, it becomes very competitive, and once people become highly competitive they are driven to do strange things.'[22]

Drug-company-sponsored clinical trials of drugs (studies in which drugs are tested 'in the field') have also come in for criticism. The *New York Times* reported investigations into whether many company-sponsored clinical trials were, in fact, just another way of 'streaming' money to doctors. The Schering-Plough inquiry heard accusations that the company 'flooded the market with pseudo-trials' and other 'thinly disguised marketing efforts.'[23] 'No Free Lunch – UK' recently raised this issue, stating:

> . . . we are concerned by the practice of research for profit. This is often conducted in General Practice where patients agree to be included in the research for altruistic reasons, yet the doctors can receive thousands of pounds profit per patient enrolled in the study. This constitutes a direct conflict of interest and it is widespread in the UK, with some practices making £50,000 in profit per year from this work.[24]

There is another way in which drug company involvement in research exerts a not so subtle influence on the body of knowledge about ADHD, and that is the influence of the profit motive. Sam Goldstein, a clinical neurologist in the USA and a previous consultant and educational author for drug companies, has made the following point:

> The nature of our capitalist system is such that if there is a profit to be made, it is much more likely a treatment will be investigated . . . There are many good psychosocial treatments that with sufficient research would probably benefit children with ADHD. No one is going to fund them because there is no profit to be made.[25]

It seems that profit determines not only what gets investigated, but what kind of findings are shared with the general public. Read on.

Dissemination of information

Drug companies have many ways of disseminating information. Research is only one of them. Supplement publishing is another. This is a 'back-door' way of publishing reports of sponsored events that have been converted into articles by company-paid writers. The resulting papers are then published as a supplement to a journal, without ever having to be peer-reviewed in the way that usually applies to papers when they are submitted for publication. These supplements have a huge influence on opinion.

Journals, too, can be sponsored by drug companies. One such journal is *Child and Adolescent Mental Health in Primary Care*, which is sponsored by Janssen-Cilag. The journal has Andrea Bilbow, founder of the ADHD group ADDISS, on the editorial board, and the issue I have seen (volume 1, issue 3, November 2003) contains two articles on ADHD, which describe it as a 'complex neurological disorder.' One of the articles also describes the production of an information pack for schools, with 'help from a pharmaceutical company.'[26] Like most similar material, the article sees fit to attack those who are critical of ADHD (either its concept or the explosion in medication that has accompanied it):

> articles discussing methylphenidate, which have appeared in the national and local press, have done little to promote understanding of this medication and its use. Unfortunately, a number of these are ill-informed and poorly researched pieces of work that have upset many families whose children already receive medication.[27]

The journal contains Internet links to pro-ADHD websites, and information on ADHD books. It also carries a half-page advert for the forthcoming ADDISS Conference. In total, 8 of its 27 pages are devoted to ADHD. The subscription card inside has on it an advertisement for Concerta. This is unlike any other journal I have come across, but may well be one of many new-wave publications.

Drug companies also produce booklets for teachers, with titles like *A Teacher's Guide to ADHD and Methylphenidate*.[28] The booklets contain no hint that ADHD is disputed as a clinical construct, but instead use the kind of statements that imply there is a biological certainty about what it is and its origins – for example, 'ADHD is a developmental condition.' The booklet from which these quotations are taken also states that 'ADHD is not a psychological problem.' It continues with some supposedly reassuring information about medication: 'The active ingredient in the medicine has been used with success for more than 40 years' and 'It is used as part of a wide range of psychological, educational and behavioural therapies.' This last sentence is an interesting one. The experience of many clinicians and parents is that this is not the case for a great many children, for whom medication is the sole intervention (more about this later in the book). Nevertheless, it is important for the drug companies to be seen to be marketing medication as part of a 'package' of treatment for a child.

Booklets such as this one therefore usually include some behaviour management advice, which is in itself quite sound and sensible. This kind of advice lends the document a certain respectability, as it comes across more as a help manual than as a medication booklet (which, of course, is what it really is). Only when (or if) the teacher turns over the booklet will he or she see, in the bottom left-hand corner, that it is a drug company publication, produced by Celltech Pharmaceuticals.

At this point in the chapter I had wanted to include a cartoon drawing from *A Teacher's Guide to ADHD and Methylphenidate*. The cartoon (on page 22 of the booklet) shows a teacher and a pupil smiling happily as the child gets on with his work. In the background are some other happy children. The caption reads, 'He's taking the pills. Everyone's feeling better.' Unfortunately, permission to reproduce this was denied. The drawing in Figure 3.1 is my own version.

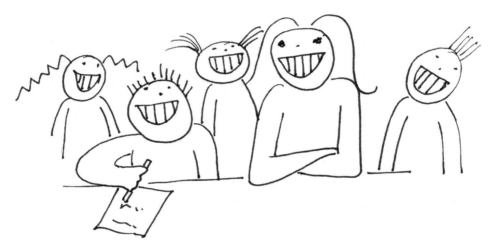

FIGURE 3.1 'We're all so much happier now that he's taking the pills!'

News groups/Internet support groups

The problem with the Internet is that it is often not clear where the information originates from. Information sites can post information that sounds authoritative, some even framing their whole newsletter as a 'research report' when it is not, like the ADHD support group, ADDISS 'report' entitled *ADHD: Paying Enough Attention?*[29] Many of these groups adopt a 'crusading' tone – a style of writing that suggests to the reader that they are having to fight for something together. Sometimes this point is made explicitly in the content. This is a psychologically powerful technique. I might not like drinking tea, but if someone tells me I'm being deprived of it (or worse still, my child is being deprived of it) and suggests that we have to band together to fight for the right to drink it, I'm likely to be right there with them! (The other thing that these groups all seem to do is to state specifically that ADHD is not the result of bad parenting. This, too, is guaranteed to get parents on side – you don't have to be a psychologist to know that this is just what we all want to hear.) In general, these information sites present themselves as parent support and advocate groups. They may indeed perform these functions, but if this is their sole aim, why do so many of them have 'sponsorship' from the drug companies? Look closely at the ADHD 'support' sites or 'news sheets' and you will find that many of them are 'sponsored' (whatever that means) by drug companies, such as Lilly*. And why do they all seem to be saying the same things?

These websites invariably promote a biological view of ADHD, and many of them include some worrying misinformation. Not only do many claim that ADHD is a 'proven' biological disorder (which it is not) with a 'definite' genetic basis (which is also unproven), but a number of websites also state that if 'the disorder' remains untreated it 'can lead to mental illness', let alone the criminal and drug-taking behaviour widely alluded to by such literature as being the fate of the 'untreated ADHD' child. Such blatant scaremongering is enough to get concerned parents running to fetch their hats and coats, with the aim of going out immediately to get some Ritalin. If it were true, I might not be far behind. But it is not. Like much of the information provided by drug companies, it is propaganda dressed up as information.

As a clinical child psychologist with considerable experience of working with children and families, I have to ask myself why it is that all of these sites seem to be saying exactly the same thing and promoting the same biological approach to children's problems. If these views were genuinely representative of the range of opinions that parents have, I can't help but think that they would be more variable. Furthermore, rather than berating the supposed shortfall in stimulant medication for children, parents would be highlighting the real lack of help for their children and themselves in terms of classroom, family and community support. Those are the comments that I hear day after day. Few parents, in my experience, come into mental health clinics on the Ritalin 'crusade.' Those that do have usually read something on the Internet the night before that has frightened them. When they have the chance to talk to someone who is genuinely interested in listening to them and helping them and their child, their relief is palpable. Most parents, thankfully, do not want to drug their children.

'Ghost writing' of medical articles

'Ghost writing' refers to the practice of authorship by someone other than the named author. In medical research, this practice has become a significant feature in recent years and has given rise to much concern. Articles are typically written by a medical writing agency, and then a potential author is sought who is prepared to put his or her name on the already prepared paper. In some instances, clinicians and researchers have discovered by accident that their names have appeared on publications without them having any knowledge of the paper in question. One such example concerned an article that was written in the names of doctors from Imperial College in London and the National Heart Institute in 2002. The *New England Journal of Medicine* was

---

* ADDISS is funded to the tune of £20,000 by Lilly, UBC Pharma and Janssen–Cilag. Foggo D. ADHD advice secretly paid for by drugs companies; www.telegraph.co.uk (accessed 9 October 2005).

forced to retract the article when one of the supposed authors, Dr Hubert Seggewiss, raised the alarm.[30]

In 2003, *The Observer* reported the experience of David Healy, a researcher at the University of Wales who was studying the negative effects of antidepressants. Healy showed the newspaper reporter, Antony Barnett, an email he had received from a drug manufacturer's representative. It read as follows: 'In order to reduce your workload to a minimum, we have had our ghost writer produce a first draft based on your published work.' Attached was a 12-page paper, prepared for presentation at a forthcoming conference. Although Healy had never seen this article before, his name appeared as the sole author. Since he believed that the paper reviewed the drug in question rather too favourably, he suggested some changes. This led to a reply from the company, suggesting that he had overlooked some 'commercially important' points. *The Observer* notes that the ghost-written paper went on to appear at the conference, as well as in a psychiatric journal, in its original form – under another doctor's name.[31]

In the same *Observer* article, we learn more about how these research 'partnerships' between researchers and the drug companies really work. For example, consider the case of Dr Aubrey Blumsohn, a senior lecturer and bone specialist at Sheffield University. Dr Blumsohn was carrying out research with the drug company Procter and Gamble into the osteoporosis drug, Actonel. In 2003, he alerted the *Journal of Bone and Mineral Research* to his concerns about some of the research published in his name, alleging that he had not been allowed to see the full analysis of the research data before the findings were written up. He wrote to the journal in November 2004, stating that 'I am the first author on both abstracts, and have serious concerns about the analysis which has been presented in my name, as first author. Is there a mechanism for comment or dissociation?'[32]

Nothing happened. Only after *The Observer* and the *Times Higher Educational Supplement* raised the issue did something happen. The journal agreed to investigate Dr Blumsohn's concerns. Unfortunately, something else occurred – Dr Blumsohn was suspended from his post at the university in September 2004, on grounds of misconduct, after talking to journalists and professional bodies about his concerns.[33]

Two years later, on 26 February 2006, *The Observer* reported that in response to their investigation a 'bill of rights' was being published by Procter and Gamble, a drugs giant. This sets out the rights of researchers to have access to all data that are relevant to their work, to enable them to 'confirm the accuracy of statements and conclusions published with them as co-authors.' Unfortunately, the article did not say whether Dr Blumsohn has been reinstated. I hope he has been.

Amazingly, recent reports suggest that *almost half* of all articles published in journals are by ghost writers.[34] There is a particular problem in the field of psychiatry, where ghost writing is increasing. Fortunately, some people are having the courage to speak out. One of these is Susanna Rees, who was until 2002 an editorial assistant for a medical writing agency. Rees described how her role had included the meticulous removal of any information that might reveal the true origins of the research. Her experiences concerned her sufficiently for her to post a letter on the website of the *British Medical Journal*, in which she stated:

Medical writing agencies go to great lengths to disguise the fact that the papers they ghost write and submit to journals and conferences are ghost written on behalf of pharmaceutical companies and not by the named authors.[35]

Dr Richard Smith, Editor of the *British Journal of Medicine*, is described in this same *Observer* article as admitting that ghost writing is a 'very big problem.' According to Smith, 'We are being hoodwinked by the drug companies.'[35]

Nowadays, we not only have ghost writers to contend with but also *ghost actors*. These are called in because the supposed authors of a paper are not sufficiently familiar with it to do their own presenting at major meetings. Either that or the event is judged to be insufficiently prestigious to warrant a real presence. At such times in come the ghost actors (usually medical writers), who present the research. Few people, if any, would know that they are not the real thing. If they did, they would probably assume that the presenter was part of the research team – perhaps a doctoral student.

Funding for pro-drug patient and carer groups

Drug companies often provide funding for patient groups to give their campaigns a higher profile. In doing so, they successfully create the impression of public demand, whereas in fact this demand has been deliberately cultivated by the drug companies themselves. Patient groups attract a lot of attention from the media and sometimes include celebrity members. Their funding by the drug companies ensures their promotion of the biological view of mental health problems – which is, of course, the drug companies' aim.

One of the best known of these groups is CHADD. The acronym CHADD stands for Children and Adults with Attention Deficit Disorder. Set up in the USA in 1987, the group is fiercely pro–ADHD, and seeks to promote a biological 'explanation' of ADHD and its treatment by stimulant medication. CHADD also runs national 'information campaigns' and engages in lobbying that vigorously opposes any proposals to restrict the prescribing of stimulants. CHADD acknowledges that a fifth of its funding is from the drug companies.[36] As you might expect, CHADD is very selective about the information that it chooses to disseminate.

For example, in 2002, Dr William Pelham, a former member of the scientific advisory board for McNeil Pharmaceuticals, which markets Concerta, received the CHADD Hall of Fame Award for his research work on ADHD. He was interviewed by the organisation's magazine, *Attention!* However, CHADD tried to suppress the interview, eventually publishing an edited version. The reason for this was that Pelham had highlighted the limitations of stimulant medication and had said that psychosocial treatments should be the treatment of first choice in ADHD. He has since stated:

> In recent years, I have come to believe that the individuals who advocate most strongly in favour of medication – both from the professional community, including the National Institute for Mental Health, and those from advocacy groups, including CHADD – have major and undisclosed conflicts of interest with the pharmaceutical companies that deal with ADHD products.[37]

Prior to his interview for *Attention!*, Pelham had for several years hosted a conference on children's mental health. This had been supported by educational grants from the drug companies McNeil (which produces Concerta) and Shire Pharmaceuticals (Adderall). Following publication of the article, this support was withdrawn.

The drug company Novartis (which produces Ritalin) and CHADD have together released material that promotes ADHD as a proven 'neurobiological disability', stating that stimulants work by 'correcting for a neurochemical imbalance.' As we have already seen, this is *only a hypothesis*, not a proven fact. Is it ethical therefore to produce material such as this, *which states as fact things that are simply theories?* More important still, is it ethical to do so when you know that what is being categorically stated is under dispute, not only in the public but also in the professional arena?

Some people think not. Their response was to bring charges against Novartis of over-promotion of ADHD and Ritalin and of collusion with the American Psychiatric Association to create an overly broad diagnostic category of ADHD. Given the widespread criticism of the subjectivity and over-inclusiveness of the *DSM* ADHD criteria, you might find it interesting that the lawsuits were withdrawn, after being ruled 'insufficiently specific.' The law is not without its sense of irony, it seems.

Political lobbying and direct funding of political bodies

The political lobbying activities of the drug companies, both in Europe and in North America, are well organised and effective. This ensures that they have influence on and access to policy makers. In comparison, the public health lobby's influence is minute. In the USA there are more pharmaceutical industry lobbyists than Congress members – a somewhat strange situation.[38]

The drug companies are major contributors to political parties on both sides of the Atlantic. In the USA, contributions peaked in 2002, presumably in line with the election campaign, with a whopping US$ 29.5 million (contributions are now down again to about US$ 18 million). This equates to a split between Republicans and Democrats of roughly 65% to 35%, respectively. This level tends to remain fairly constant.

Like me, you might reason that one of the main motives for giving money to political parties is to gain access (otherwise, why do it?). Most of us would go further. We might hazard a guess that when someone does this, they presumably expect something in return. Experience suggests that they usually get it, too. For example, in the UK, consider the case of Paul Drayson of the drug company PowderJect, who in 2004 was given a peerage. One month later he donated £500,000 to the governing Labour party. Immediately prior to this, PowderJect had been awarded a substantial government contract.[39]

Regulatory agencies are also not immune to drug company influence. In the UK, the Medicines and Healthcare products Regulatory Agency (MHRA) is the regulatory body that governs the production of medication. It is one of only two European medicine regulators wholly funded by the pharmaceutical industry.

In the USA, a review of financial disclosure requirements for National Institutes of Health (NIH) personnel was announced in December 2003 by the NIH itself, in an attempt to increase public confidence. This followed an article in *The Los Angeles Times* which gave details of hundreds of consultation payments from biomedical companies to NIH employees.[40] Before you draw breath in horror, you might like to remind yourself that a similar disclosure process has not yet occurred in the UK.

Shaping views on mental health

As we have seen, the influence of the drug companies on prescribing is extensive and deliberate. Over the years, this has had a very significant effect on how mental health problems are viewed and treated. In many cases, drug company 'wisdom' has become the accepted wisdom and has been incorporated into clinical practice guidelines. In her article, 'Is Psychiatry for Sale?', Joanna Moncrieff tells us that in 2002, 87% of clinical practice guidelines were reported to have had some interaction with the pharmaceutical industry, and over a third of those involved had served as either consultants or employees of drug companies.[41] How can we be sure that these recommendations and guidelines are in our best interests, rather than those of the drug companies? The answer is that we can't.

CHAPTER 4

The rise and rise of biological psychiatry

Psychiatrists have been increasingly targeted by drug companies in recent years and this has led, predictably one might say, not only to more prescribing but to a growth in 'biological psychiatry' and the 'disease' model of mental health. This is the school of thought that views mental health problems as diseases that are caused by underlying biological processes – just like any other disease. And just like physical diseases, their 'treatment' consists of medication to correct whatever biological defect the person is deemed to have. Thus the relationship between psychiatrists and drug companies has become one of perfect reflexivity – put simply, each drives the other. As more 'disorders' become identified and as diagnostic categories become wider and more inclusive, more drugs are prescribed, greater profits are made and more drug companies can engage in research activities which, in turn, influence the search for evidence of new diagnostic categories and new drugs. And so the cycle goes on (and on, and on . . .).

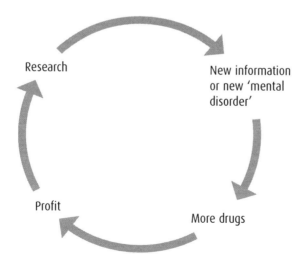

FIGURE 4.1 Perpetual motion: how biological psychiatry and the drug industry work in perfect harmony.

This kind of vicious circle leads to the development of drugs that we neither want nor need. Often referred to as 'me too' drugs, these are constant updates or copies of rival best-sellers that offer nothing new. Nevertheless, the drug companies market them as more up-to-date versions of existing drugs, and of course they are usually more expensive.

In order to make sense, the disease model *must* promote medical solutions, and it does so in a way that exaggerates the advantages and minimises the disadvantages of drug use. This is not only highly relevant to all of us who are, after all, potential consumers of these drugs, but it should also remind us of previous experiences of 'wonder drugs' which have turned out to be anything but that. Two of the most popular families of drugs in recent years have been the benzodiazepines and the antidepressants. The literature suggests that we are not learning from experience. Let us remind ourselves.

The benzodiazepines

Some of you might remember the benzodiazepines. I certainly do. They are still around, of course, but not in the quantities they used to be. During the mid-1980s, I was an assistant psychologist in the Midlands, working in community settings with adults (mostly women) who had problems with anxiety. Many of them had a diagnosis of agoraphobia. All of the people whom I saw during my clinical placement were already on medication when they were sent to us for help. Many of them were fairly long-term users of tranquillisers and sleeping tablets that belonged to the family of drugs known as benzodiazepines (*see* Box 4.1). The most popular of these drugs in my particular client group were diazepam (Valium) and lorazepam (Ativan).

As an assistant psychologist, my task was to help with desensitisation – the process whereby people with phobias are helped to cope by gradual exposure to the feared situation or object. Part of my role was to teach relaxation and to help those I worked with to develop some psychological coping strategies that would help them to regain the confidence to venture out into the world again.*

I had an excellent supervisor (Barbara Baxter), and the people I tried to help did well. However, when they tried to reduce their medication, they found that their symptoms started to return, and were sometimes even worse then before. Unless you have witnessed the distress caused by overwhelming physiological symptoms of sufficient severity to cause fainting, and have held the violently trembling hands of people suffering hallucinations, delusions and feelings of absolute dread, you can't imagine what these people endured. I was aware of others who had previously given up their attempts to wean themselves off their drugs, so severe were the effects that they experienced. Many, of course, assumed that their illness had returned and that their distressing experiences were 'proof' that they still needed their tranquillisers. Their doctors tended to see it this way, too, and often increased their patients' prescriptions.

---

* Clinical psychology training is long and arduous, requiring the would-be clinical psychologist to gain 'field' experience, sometimes for several years, between their first degree in psychology and their clinical doctorate. In the UK, this time is most often spent as an assistant psychologist, working in the NHS.

They were wrong. What I was witnessing were the effects of what we now know as benzodiazepine addiction.

The wonder drugs

Benzodiazepines were the wonder drugs of the 1970s. They were prescribed for problems such as stress, insomnia and anxiety, including phobic anxiety such as the agoraphobia experienced by so many of the people whom I met and got to know through working with them. Only later did we start to realise that the 'cure' was far worse than the complaint had ever been. Unfortunately, many people continued to be prescribed this group of medications. Some of them have taken benzodiazepines for up to 30 or 40 years. According to Dr Reg Peart, in his submission to the Select Committee on Health Inquiry in June 1999, 90% of users of these drugs become addicted within 1 to 2 years. Dr Peart was himself addicted to Valium for 15 years, something he described as 'chemical rape of the mind, body and soul.'[1]

BOX 4.1 The benzodiazepines

In 1963, approval was given for the first available benzodiazepine, which was diazepam (Valium), to be used for the treatment of anxiety. Two years later, nitrazepam (Mogadon) was introduced to treat sleep problems. Benzodiazepines replaced barbiturates, which had previously been the drugs of choice for such problems, and began to be widely prescribed during the 1960s and 1970s. The new drugs were introduced as being safer, as they had a lower potential for abuse and relatively fewer adverse reactions. They also had fewer interaction effects and, unlike the barbiturates, it was not so easy to take a fatal overdose of benzodiazepines. Only later was it realised that these were not the 'wonder drugs' they had first appeared to be. Not only do they have adverse side-effects, but they are also addictive and cause *iatrogenic disease* (i.e. disease resulting from treatment).

Benzodiazepine withdrawal syndrome is characterised by insomnia, anxiety, confusion, tremor, perspiration, loss of appetite, perceptual disorders, delusions and, occasionally, fits. These symptoms may sometimes be indistinguishable from the original symptoms for which the person sought help. Benzodiazepines are also the largest group of recreationally used drugs.[2] One member of this family of drugs that has been withdrawn in some countries is flunitrazepam (Rohypnol), often referred to as the 'date-rape drug.'

Benzodiazepine dependence is now widely recognised. In 1988, the UK Committee on Safety of Medicines recommended that their use be limited to 'short-term relief' of anxiety symptoms, which it defined as '2 to 4 weeks only.' It added that the use of such drugs to treat short-term or 'mild' anxiety is 'inappropriate and unsuitable.'[3] The National Service Framework (NSF) for mental health, published in 1999, recommended that benzodiazepines should be used for no more than 2 to 4 weeks for severe and disabling anxiety.[4] In 2004, the Chief Medical Officer's update from the Department of Health 'reminded' doctors of this earlier guidance, citing Department of Health data that suggested patients were still receiving long-term treatment with these drugs.[5] Most of these are older adults – over half of all UK prescriptions for the three commonest benzodiazepines are dispensed to people over the age of 65 years.*

The antidepressants

Antidepressants are taken by billions of people across the world. In the USA alone, it was calculated in 2003 that over 28 million people had started taking Prozac since it was first launched in 1987, while 45 million Americans had started taking either Paxil or Zoloft since they were launched in 1992.[6] Together, this represents *more than the entire population of some countries, including the UK.*

Despite the popularity of antidepressants, a number of studies have questioned their effectiveness, suggesting that there is little difference between antidepressants and placebo ('dummy') drugs.[7] This has prompted some researchers to suggest that antidepressants have been touted by the drug companies as being much more effective than they actually are.

Recent evidence has tended to contradict earlier views that these drugs were safe and without side-effects. For instance, it is known that the commonest group of antidepressants, namely the SSRIs (*see* Box 4.2), often cause sexual dysfunction, which can persist long after medication has been stopped. Some patients report severe side-effects, particularly with paroxetine (Paxil or Seroxat), and some lethal reactions to another group of antidepressants, known as monoamine oxidase inhibitors (MAOIs), have occurred. It has also been suggested that some antidepressants may cause dependence.

SEROXAT MUST NOT BE USED FOR TREATMENT OF CHILDREN WITH DEPRESSION

Department of Health Press Release: Tuesday 10 June, 2003. Reference number: 2003/0223

New expert advice recommends that the drug Seroxat (paroxetine) is not used to treat children and teenagers under the age of 18 years for depressive illness, said Professor Alasdair Breckenridge, Chairman of the Medicines and Healthcare Products Regulatory Agency.

New data, received within the last two weeks, has been evaluated and considered by the Committee on Safety of Medicines (CSM) and its Expert Working Group on SSRIs. It shows that there is an increase in the rate of self-harm and potentially suicidal behaviour in this age group, when Seroxat is used for depressive illness. It has become clear that the benefits of Seroxat in children for the treatment of depressive illness do not outweigh these risks.

Ironically, it has recently been recognised that some antidepressants have side-effects *that make self-harm and suicide more likely.* Amidst growing concern, in 2003 the Department of Health in the UK issued a press release stating that the antidepressant paroxetine (Seroxat) must not be used for the treatment of children. This was followed in 2004 by a public health advisory statement by the Food and Drug Administration in the USA, in which manufacturers of antidepressant drugs were asked to include

---

* *Source:* Department of Health 2002 data for England; www.benzo.org.uk

in their labelling a warning statement that recommends close observation of adult and paediatric patients for worsening depression and the emergence of 'suicidality.' This followed allegations that emerging information about the increased risk of suicide and self-harm among young people taking certain antidepressants was being suppressed.[8]

BOX 4.2 The antidepressants

Antidepressants were discovered as a 'by-product' of tuberculosis research in the 1950s, but were not used clinically until the 1960s. The first widely used antidepressant was imipramine, which is known as a tricylic antidepressant (TCA). Other types of drug, known as monoamine oxidase inhibitors (MAOIs), were developed at almost the same time. Both of these types of drugs caused unpleasant side-effects, such as sedation. There were also safety and toxicity concerns, as well as potentially dangerous interaction effects (caused when drugs are combined with other drugs). From the 1970s onwards, new types of drugs known as selective serotonin reuptake inhibitors (SSRIs) began to be developed. The first of these was fluoxetine (Prozac). These newer, safer drugs were tolerated well by patients, thus allowing them to be treated in the primary care setting rather than having to be referred to a psychiatrist, as had previously been the case.

As with the benzodiazepines, over time there has been growing concern about these drugs. Newborn babies of mothers who had been taking antidepressants while pregnant began to be born with severe withdrawal symptoms which included shaking, convulsions, irritability and abnormal crying. The drug that posed the greatest risk was identified as Seroxat.[9] Other research has warned of the increased risk of stillbirths and birth defects.[10] In June 2004, GlaxoSmithKline, the London-based Anglo-American pharmaceuticals group, was accused of 'fraudulently suppressing research that suggested that Paxil was ineffective and unsafe in treating children, possibly causing them to commit suicide.'[11,12] In 2003, *The Observer* reported that Prozac was being taken in such large quantities that it could now be found in drinking water throughout the UK.[13]

The use of antidepressants over the past 40 years has increased markedly, and this is reflected in increases in prescriptions for children, including very young children.[14]

Antidepressants, like the benzodiazepines before them, are creating concern and controversy. These are only two groups of drugs that have been hailed as new 'breakthrough' drugs in mental health. It seems as though we are indeed not learning the lessons of history.

Blind faith

It does seem remarkable that we continue taking 'what the doctor orders' despite the latest 'breakthrough' drugs proving, with depressing regularity, to be actually harmful. We continue to trust in prescribed medicines despite losing our faith in just about everything else. Why is this?

One reason is that medical science, and the pharmaceutical industry in particular, has taken the credit for the huge improvements in health and longevity over the past century – a medical miracle that most of us are in awe of. Although it is true that very significant benefits have been brought about by certain drugs, it is also the case that the health of most individuals in industrialised countries has been vastly improved by developments such as clean water, better hygiene and good nutrition. We live longer because of our lifestyles, and we are healthier because we tend not to become ill in the first place.[15]

Another reason for our continued trust in medicine might be that it really is a matter of faith. We want to believe that medicine can save us. For most of us, this includes, perhaps second only to surgery, the hope of newer and better drugs. Nothing is so certain for us all than increasing frailty and probable illness as we grow older. Like most of you, I also hope for a cure for Alzheimer's before it gets me.

This type of thinking promotes a 'blind faith' in drugs that is not only undeserved but dangerous. Unfortunately, it also seems to govern the kind of attitudes we have to drugs that are given to us as 'cures' for psychological distress. This has required a large leap of faith. In this case, however, we didn't jump – we were pushed.

Influence on thinking

The drug companies have had a key role in developing and maintaining a narrow biological approach to the understanding of mental health problems as 'diseases' that need medical treatment. The most important consequence of this has been that this view has become so dominant that it leaves little or no room for others. So pervasive has its influence been that the biological (medical) model is now accepted as 'the truth' in a way that relegates non-medical approaches to the fringes of mental health. My professional experience is that the past 20 or so years have seen mental health 'hijacked' by a different kind of psychiatry from that which I knew as a student and during my early years of practice as a clinical psychologist. In those days, many psychiatrists whom I met had also chosen to train as psychotherapists and family therapists. Their medical training was, in a sense, an *added ingredient* of their mental health skills. Nowadays, the balance is much more likely to be tipped the other way. I can't emphasise enough the part played by ADHD in bringing about this change in the field of children's mental health. It has been a major contributory factor in bringing about a psychiatry that is, for the most part, far less concerned with the mind than it used to be, and much more preoccupied with (what it imagines to be) the workings of the brain.

In this kind of psychiatry, our experiences – however complex – are explained away as simple biochemical responses. It is our *biochemistry* that is responsible for the way we feel – never mind the quality of our relationships, our upbringing or the social and cultural contexts in which we live. This explanation of mental health is now established as a thread of understanding that runs through every aspect of our lives. It has taken years to weave, but is now so beautifully integrated at every level that it is viewed almost as heresy to argue with it.

Perhaps most importantly of all, this biological hegemony has social and political consequences. After all, if a person's problem is a 'disease' or 'malfunction' in their brain, that makes life easy. We don't have to think about the social aspects of that person's life at all, or how these might contribute to the development of mental ill health. We don't need to think about the political issues that play an important part in maintaining people in conditions that undermine good mental health. We don't need to think about how their difficulties are identified, classified and diagnosed. Put bluntly, it suits us to have mental health problems classified as diseases. It might also suit those in positions of political power to have a dominant model of mental health that allows them to abdicate responsibility while at the same time enabling them to show publicly the requisite degree of concern.

Influence that goes right to the top . . .

With these things in mind, it is of concern that high-level partnerships with drug companies are now beginning to impact on practice guidelines and government policy in the UK.[16] For some time it has been the case that some doctors have had a significant influence on local and national healthcare policy. So perhaps it was only a matter of time before the drug companies began to forge the kind of partnerships that would influence decision making at the very top. Having done this, they are now in a position to steer all-important healthcare decision making that affects every individual. This really does represent integration of the biological model at the highest level, and it hints at the kind of influences on our lives that have previously only been imagined as science fiction.

Joanna Moncrieff, in her paper entitled 'Is psychiatry for sale?', warns of drug company influence on central government policy in the UK through recently established government bodies. She lists these as follows:

- the pharmaceutical industry competitiveness task force
- the industry strategy group
- partnerships with health service bodies
- the National Institute for Mental Health England (NIMHE)
- the pharmaceutical industry represented by the Association of the British Pharmaceutical Industry (ABPI).

Her concern – and it is a concern shared by many health workers – is that as a result of these partnerships, drug treatment will be overemphasised (and presumably other non-medical approaches will be underemphasised). She comments on these projects and the NIMHE statement that it expects drug industry partnerships to become routine in the development and implementation of mental health policy, pointing out that:

> incorporating the industry into the fabric of the health service in this way increases its influence enormously and may make it very difficult to identify and resist commercial pressures. There seems to be little acknowledgement that there might be conflicts of interest between the aims of industry and those of a public service.[17]

TMAP: a 'nice' partnership

In trying to understand some of the reasoning that has brought us to this position, it is helpful to look back, particularly to the precursors to some of these 'partnerships.' One of these antecedents was the Texas Medication Algorithm Project.

In 1995, the Texas Medication Algorithm Project, otherwise known as TMAP, was launched to develop medication algorithms for mental disorders in the Texan public health sector. Initially funded by Janssen Pharmaceuticals (Johnson and Johnson), these made recommendations about drug treatment for a range of mental health problems, the earliest one being schizophrenia. TMAP was recommended by the 'New Freedom Commission on Mental Health' set out by US President George W Bush, and has been extended to other states, where it has been very influential. Some US states can insist that the TMAP algorithms are followed.

There are some uncomfortable political ties to drug companies that call into question the motivation behind drug recommendations and even the process itself. Critics have suggested that the system amounts to little more than a marketing scheme. There is an obvious benefit to drug companies of their drugs being identified in the medication algorithm, especially when newer, more expensive drugs become introduced and are recommended over older ones. For example, after TMAP made the new Eli Lilly drug, *olanzapine*, the first-line treatment for schizophrenia, it became Lilly's top-selling drug, grossing US$ 4.2 billion (£2.35 billion) worldwide in 2003. Who knows whether the fact that George Bush senior used to be on the Lilly board of directors influenced this decision, or what part was played by George W Bush appointing Lilly's Chief Executive Officer, Sidney Taurel, to a seat on the Homeland Security Council – or indeed what was behind the total contribution of US$ 1.6 million made by Eli Lilly in 2000, 82% of which went to the Republican party.[18]

Those who have spoken out against the ways in which drug companies seek to influence TMAP receive a powerful message. In 2004, the *British Medical Journal* reported on 'whistleblowers' Stefan Kruszeuski and Allen Jones. Jones was an inspector with the Pennsylvania office of the Inspector General. He was sacked after he revealed that money and other 'perks' were given to key officials by drug companies keen to influence the content of the drug algorithms. Psychiatrist Stefan Kruszeuski, another Pennsylvania official investigating fraud, was also fired for revealing corrupt practices.[19]

Screening for all

In 2004, US$ 20 million were put aside by Congress to implement the findings of the 'New Freedom Commission on Mental Health', which made the recommendation of routine screening of 'consumers of all ages' for mental health problems. This included schoolchildren and pre-schoolers. One of the results of this has been 'Teen Screen', a programme to assess US schoolchildren for mental illness. 'Teen Screen' has raised concerns that a cohort of perfectly ordinary, healthy young people are at risk of being classified as mentally ill, like the 15-year-old daughter of Mike and Teresa Rhodes, who was screened in her school in Indiana and diagnosed with obsessive-compulsive disorder and social anxiety disorder. Once a child has been diagnosed, prescribed medical treatment follows, with parental concerns overridden by mental health officials if necessary. Mr and Mrs Rhodes have mounted the first legal challenge against 'Teen Screen', but it continues to be rolled out and there are still plans to go ahead with whole population screening for 'mental illness.'

NICE or not so nice?

Despite criticisms of TMAP, the UK has not been far behind in following suit. The National Institute for Clinical Excellence (NICE) describes itself as an NHS agency, set up in 1999 to make recommendations in England and Wales about treatments and medical procedures. Most appraisals undertaken by NICE concern pharmaceuticals. From the start it has been controversial. One of the first things it did was to recommend against prescribing the influenza vaccine, Relenza, in October 1999. This position was changed soon afterwards, following criticism from the drug industry. There have been a number of similar controversial decisions.

Commentators have remarked that the recommendations made by NICE are remarkably similar to TMAP and earlier drug-company-sponsored guidelines. Like TMAP, recommendations have been drawn up by 'expert' consensus, rather than through evidence of effectiveness. It has been claimed that those responsible for drawing up the algorithms have extensive financial connections with the drug companies. One-third of the panels have declared links, and up to 70% of those sitting on panels are believed to be affected. In one case every single member of the panel was paid by the company whose drug ended up being recommended.[20]

With regard to antipsychotic drugs, a number of writers have commented on the similarities between the NICE guidelines and those drawn up by TMAP and other drug companies. Like TMAP, NICE recommends the use of newer antipsychotics over older ones, *despite its own acknowledgement that there is no evidence base for this*. It has been pointed out that the older antipsychotics continue to be safer and more reliable. Adherence to the guidelines could therefore be detrimental to patient care.[21]

As Taylor and Giles have cautioned in their critique of such 'advice', the NICE guidelines present a further dilemma for practitioners, as it may prove difficult to 'opt out' of them, given their endorsement by the government and the healthcare system. Those who find themselves practising outside the guidelines are likely to have to justify their decision making in a way that can demonstrate effectiveness, including cost-effectiveness[22] – never mind what they think is best for their client. This is a significant departure from the principle of clinical autonomy.

The same authors also highlight the fact that by 'recommending' newer drugs as they are developed, NICE has a further important impact on the NHS. It effectively introduces the philosophy of ever increasing costs while 'capping' expectations about health improvements. This is important because, as we all know, there is limited funding within mental health, and therefore any increased expenditure on drugs means that other areas will have *less* money spent on them. This inevitably leaves other mental health 'treatments' under-resourced, leading to less rather than more patient choice, and little development of proven, effective therapies. Next time you or a member of your family are told that you will have to wait up to a year to see a therapist, you will know why.

In the UK, the Critical Psychiatry Network (an organisation of psychiatrists) has expressed concern about the possible influence of drug companies on government bodies, especially NIMHE and NICE. This view was endorsed by a number of those involved in the House of Commons inquiry into the influence of the pharmaceutical companies – for example, by Dr Doug Naysmith, MP for Bristol North West, who commented that 'we have received a large body of evidence from various sources which argues that the pharmaceutical industry wields extensive influence on healthcare policy and systems in this country.' Strangely enough, it seems that just about everyone is worried about this relationship – except for the government, that is, who deny seeing any dangers.

There is a saying, much used by family therapists, which I think originated in China. It goes something like this: 'Only the fish have no understanding that it is *water* they are swimming in.'

NICE and ADHD

Unfortunately, NICE seems to have accepted, remarkably uncritically, the idea that ADHD is a bona-fide brain disease. It regurgitates some of the well-known propaganda about ADHD, including the following: 'Heredity aspects, neuroimaging data and responses to pharmacotherapeutic agents support the suggestion that ADHD has a biological component.' The guideline is expected in 2008.

Accountability

The activities and conduct of the drug companies are coming under increasing scrutiny by the media in many countries, and this is perceived by most as being a positive development. It seems unlikely that there will be any reform of current practices without this kind of pressure. There have been other kinds of scrutiny, too, such as that undertaken by the UK Parliamentary Health Committee, which has examined evidence on the influence of the drug industry on the wider healthcare sector. The committee has expressed concern on a number of fronts, mostly centring on the need for greater openness and accountability. However, it should be remembered that Parliamentary Committees have no power to implement recommendations (in this case, 48 of them). Their job is to advise the government, whose ministers we can only hope will pretty quickly develop a sense of what it is they are swimming in (and at this point some of you might be thinking it's not water).

The conflict of interest in the relationship between the drug companies and the medical profession lies in the propensity for mutual gain that is not necessarily in keeping with public health interests. This reason alone should raise doubts about the kinds of partnerships that currently exist. As Moncrieff cautions, the drug companies' *raison d'être* is, of course, to make a profit, and although in a business sense this might be understandable, in the context of medicine it is not.[23]

There is a strong and sensible argument for the view that the NHS should not be in business with the drug companies under any circumstances, and furthermore that it should not be allowing doctors to act as partners to these companies in their primary aim of profiteering, as seems to be the case. This constitutes far too much of a risk to service users. Dr Reg Peart, in his submission to the Select Committee on Health Inquiry into Benzodiazepines, suggests that these relationships seriously threaten the old medical precept, 'first do no harm.' He is right. To remind ourselves, here's a translation from Hippocrates:

> Declare the past, diagnose the present, foretell the future; practice these acts. As to diseases, make a habit of two things – to help, or at least to do no harm.[*]

---

[*] The phrase 'first do no harm' comes from Hippocrates' *Epidemics, Book One* (section XI), not from the Hippocratic Oath, as is commonly believed.

CHAPTER 5

What's happening to our children?

ADHD has been described as a good example of a situation where the cure was invented before the problem. Apart from politics, it's hard to find a situation where you might do things in this kind of way, first deciding on what you want to do and then – working backwards – finding a reason to do it.

Not only has this kind of backwards chaining happened with stimulant medication and ADHD, but we also seem to have allowed ourselves to be persuaded that it is perfectly all right to 'treat' a condition whose very existence is still being debated among experts. The information reviewed suggests that there are two main reasons for this: first, the aggressive marketing tactics of the drug companies, who have vigorously promoted ADHD as a biological disorder, and secondly, the increasingly close partnership between the drug companies and psychiatry. This partnership has in turn had a strong influence on how psychiatry has developed, and has served to expand and legitimise its biological identity.

However, it would be too simple to blame the drug companies and their influence on psychiatrists for the massive increase in the number of children labelled as having ADHD in recent years. We are all involved in this. To put it bluntly, the drug companies simply couldn't do it without our help.

How we have all helped to create the ADHD epidemic

There are many different strands to the ADHD epidemic and many ways in which we have all contributed to the present–day scenario. To discover how we have done this, we need to start by taking a closer look at our modern day-to-day lives.

Modern life is rubbish*

People are generally uneasy about the rapid changes in living that have taken place over the last 40 to 50 years. Put simply, we are not quite sure that we like this. Although many changes have proved advantageous, there is a general sense that what passes for progress, although leaving many people materially better off, has meant huge trade-offs

---

* In 1993, the UK band *Blur* released an album entitled *Modern Life is Rubbish* – echoing, it seemed, the thoughts of the time and a tendency for us all to look back with nostalgia to better times. But some people think it might be true.

in other respects. Increased prosperity has brought with it enormous social change, to the extent that twenty-first-century family life does not resemble anything like our grandparents' or even our parents' lives. As the pace of change has quickened, so unease has grown. Sometimes it's hard to know what the unease is about.

Modern life means that social behaviour is no longer driven by obligation, custom or practice but by *choice*. In theory this is great. In reality it means that each individual or couple has to define for themselves the parameters of their lives, their relationships and their family. This is not an easy task. For one thing, there is no template for family life, as there used to be, so it can be difficult to know whether what you're doing is right or wrong. As if this wasn't hard enough, the context for all of these life decisions is no longer the extended family or neighbourhood. Both of these, for most people, are things of the past. Nowadays we look to the 'expert culture' for advice on what we should be doing. This applies most of all in areas like child-rearing, education, health and social care. All of these areas are now the business of 'experts.' Predictably, this leaves us feeling helpless (and maybe more than a little hopeless). It also leaves us ready to hand over our responsibility for all kinds of things to the 'experts' (whoever they are). It comes as no surprise, then, that today's parents have found themselves feeling deskilled.

There is something else at work here. What modern life gives us is the sense that if we pay for something it should work. The biggest trade-off of all is that we willingly collude with some of the things that we are uneasy about in return for a life that offers material comforts and increased prosperity. When things work it seems like a good trade-off. When there is a hint that they might not work, we get angry and confused:[*] 'Hang on, I paid for this. I work hard nine to five for this. My life is organised around this. It should work.' It might not be such a bad argument, in itself – unless we apply it to our children.

Why are parents anxious?

Modern life is shot through with fear and anxiety, much of which relates to our children. Being a parent means that we naturally spend a lot of our time worrying about whether we are doing it right. When we are not doing this, we are probably worrying about the world 'out there' and what it's doing to our children. We only have to open our newspaper or switch on our TV and there will probably be something that will add to our fears – antisocial and violent behaviour on the streets, escalating levels of drug and alcohol misuse, rising levels of teenage pregnancy, behaviour in school, behaviour out of school, children who are 'uncontrollable', unteachable or unreachable. The natural 'angst' of parents everywhere has been amplified by the kind of focus that suggests there is something biologically wrong with our children. (This comes hand in hand, by the way, with film and television stereotypes that give us unreal expectations – not just about our children but also about ourselves.)

Modern society gives us many good reasons to be dissatisfied. It 'primes' us to be concerned about our children while at the same time furnishing us with certain ideas

---

[*] This idea is a theme in Robert M Pirsig's *Zen and the Art of Motorcycle Maintenance*. London: Corgi; 1976.

and expectations about children, parents and family life. It also provides us with a strong sense of where to take these concerns – to an 'expert' who can fix them. The fix, of course, is usually a medical one.

You might be forgiven for thinking at this point that our children serve as useful points of projection of all our worries about the kinds of societies we have created. There is doubtless some truth in this, but it is not the whole story.

Why do parents worry about ADHD?

Many parents and teachers report that children are unable to pay attention and concentrate 'properly', and many more complain of children having so-called 'behaviour problems.' This does not mean that they have ADHD (and when mental health workers like myself see them, this is usually quickly confirmed).

Parents come to see me for many reasons. The majority of times they are perfectly adequate parents who want to do the best for their child and just need reassurance that everything they are doing is right. Often something has happened that has knocked their confidence out of kilter, or for some reason their normal coping threshold has been lowered. Sometimes a life change has plunged them or their child into crisis. The end result is the same – what they usually do does not seem to be working. Fortunately, for 'perfectly adequate parents' (which most of us are) and 'usually OK kids' (which most of them are) it is not too difficult to find, or rediscover, a way of coping with most problems.

In recent years, however, things have started to become very different. Where parents previously looked for help, advice or support, some now arrive forearmed with information on ADHD that suggests a different kind of answer altogether. There is definitely much more concern nowadays about children's behaviour and particularly about ADHD, with many parents asking directly 'Could he have ADHD?' Sometimes their concern has been raised by something that has been reported on television or in the news. Often it has been something they have discovered on the Internet. Some of this material is alarming. Much of it, as we have seen, presents ADHD as an incurable brain disorder. Some of it suggests that if ADHD is left 'untreated', children will develop into drug addicts and/or criminals or become mentally ill.

Should parents be worried?

Are we right to be concerned about our children? The answer to this question has to be a resounding 'yes' – but not in the way that we are being told we should be.

There are some genuine concerns about children's behaviour that help to drive the ADHD phenomenon. They do this because they are – incorrectly – viewed as 'evidence' of ADHD. However, clinical as well as research experience suggests otherwise. What is most frequently called ADHD is likely to be a *mislabelling* of children's behaviours, which are often themselves adaptations to the environments in which children live and the experiences that they have. In short, children react to what happens to them. It's not rocket science. To put it bluntly, we need to be concerned about the kinds of lives our children are living.

Children rarely tell us when they are unhappy, even if they are old enough to have the language to do this. Instead *they show us*, by their behaviour, whenever they are distressed, anxious and fearful, as well as when they are happy and secure. Child experts already know a great deal about what kinds of things are harmful and damaging to children, and also what needs to be done to help them and their families and carers. It is unfortunate that, rather than addressing some of the negative influences in children's lives, some prefer to see the way children adapt to these as 'proof' that they have a 'disorder.'

If we are going to do justice to the concerns voiced by children, young people and their families, we need to be able to view their difficulties through what has been called a 'wide-angle lens.'* This means that we must be able to look beyond 'the problem' and take into account all of the things that have contributed to the life of the child or young person so far (as well as the problem). This is where the concept of the 'environment' comes in.

The importance of environment

We often hear 'environmental factors' mentioned in relation to children's mental health. And more often than not nowadays we are likely to hear them dismissed or trivialised as add-ons that exacerbate the 'real' underlying biological problems that kids have. But what do we mean when we talk about the importance of the environment in children's lives? In the way that it is meant here, the term 'environment' refers to the millions of influences on our children *from the outside*, rather than *from within* each individual child. These influences (such as family, neighbourhood or school) might seem to some negligible on their own, but when combined with hundreds and thousands of others and repeated over entire lifetimes, they have a considerable impact on the way that children feel, think and behave. Some of them have arisen from changed and changing societies, families and lifestyles. Some have not.

In general, children's environments have changed dramatically in recent years. As a result, their experiences of growing up differ enormously from those of previous generations. There have been a number of questions raised about what might be the impact of these changes on families, and specifically on children. Some of these are worth revisiting here.

The disappearing childhood

Discuss childhood with any group of adults and the chances are the consensus will be that childhood is fast disappearing. Of course, childhood was only ever a relatively modern concept to begin with, and children as young as five used to be routinely expected to go out to work to support the family. Early twentieth-century ideas about childhood developed a mythology around the sanctity of childhood which has predominated in modern industrialised societies, sitting very uncomfortably alongside our rapidly changing, child-unfriendly societies.

---

* I am grateful to Alan Parry and Robert Doan for this metaphor, which I would like to think has informed my work since the day I read it in their book. The full reference is Parry A, Doan R. *Story Revisions: narrative therapy in the postmodern world.* New York: Guilford Press; 1994.

We have seen some important changes in the way that children are thought about as we have entered the twenty-first century and, inevitably, this translates into how they behave. We seem to have higher expectations of very young children, in terms of their behaviours and accomplishments, while at the same time the later stages of childhood have been 'stretched' into what is really a relatively new concept called 'adolescence.' One of the reasons for this has doubtless been the increasingly prohibitive cost of independence in capitalist Western cultures – young people simply do not have the resources to enable them to be fully independent. Whereas in previous times adulthood began when children left school and began to earn a wage, nowadays it is not unusual to find adults still living with their parents at the age of 30.

We tolerate children in our society as long as they behave like mini-adults – they are targeted by the fashion industry, the kiddie pop music industry and the gadget industry. They dress like little adults, are sexualised by advertising and other media, and are bombarded with advertising. Whereas in previous generations their role in life was to contribute to the economy by working, now their role is to contribute by becoming *consumers* as early as possible.

Whatever happened to play?

Modern life is characterised by a reduced scope for play. Children do not have the opportunities that their parents and grandparents did for explorative play and real-life problem solving. Instead, their parents, worried about their children's safety, expect them to *amuse themselves* with TV, games consoles and other indoor, mainly solitary activities. They expect this from a very early age. My clinical experience with families suggests that it is not unusual for children aged 4 or 5 years to be bought a games console for Christmas or a birthday. These are children who are scarcely out of nursery school, are barely toilet trained and are still struggling to develop the motor skills necessary to eat with a knife and fork. Yet they are expected to be able to amuse themselves with electronic games.

Our definition of play has also changed considerably over the years. For instance, it is common for parents to take their children to an indoor 'Play Barn' attached to a pub, and leave them in a netted adventure area to run wild. Although it might appear to the outsider that children in this environment are playing together, in fact they are not. The play is mainly solitary. This contrasts with the traditional view of play as mostly a social activity. Not too long ago, children were expected to play with their neighbourhood friends in the garden, street, field, wood or playground for most of their out-of-school time. In doing this, they not only learned to cooperate, take turns and deal with conflict, but they also learned a lot of other social rules that began to shape them as individuals.

Play is not only primarily social, but it is also something that children *learn* by playing with their parents, siblings and other children. Those of you who have read *The Secret Garden* by Frances Hodgson Burnett will remember how the brittle, sad and sickly Mary was brought to life by the garden. You might also recall how Mary didn't know how to play when she first arrived at Misselthwaite Manor, because no one had ever played with her. 'I don't play', she told the maidservant, Martha, who bought her a skipping rope and demonstrated how to use it.

One of the commonest complaints I have heard from parents who are convinced that there is something wrong with their child is 'He doesn't know how to play' or 'She just goes from one thing to another.' And yet, when I explore further, I discover that the child is tucked away somewhere apart from his or her parents, expected to just get on with it. Parents seldom *play with* their children nowadays. This is doubly sad because not only does the child miss out on learning to play, but also the adults miss out on some of the most important building blocks in forging a secure and happy relationship with their child.

Play as physical activity

The recent concerns about childhood obesity have led to a renewed focus on the amount of activity that children engage in at school. The fact is that school-age children nowadays get far less physical exercise than previous generations. Often children are transported to school, rather than taken on foot. Once there, they might find playtimes used for other things, such as extra lessons. Ironically, the active child who might get into trouble is the one who will also find him- or herself kept in at playtime as punishment. In class there is an expectation that even young children will sit still and learn. Critics contend that changing practices and expectations in classrooms have led to the normal childhood need for stimulation and activity being relabelled as abnormal, and they suggest that drugs such as Ritalin are used primarily to control or sedate 'problem' children so that they will not disrupt the class.

Does television cause ADHD?

There have been reports that there is a direct relationship between television and ADHD.[1] I have absolutely no doubt that television does *not* cause ADHD. However, I believe it to be one of many influences that in combination have a very significant impact on our children.

Television is a real tour-de-force in most people's homes, with children watching several hours per day. Media surveys suggest that sometime between their fourth and sixth birthday, nearly half of all children will acquire a television in their bedrooms.* Children are bombarded with sound and images at the rate of an image change every one or two seconds. Children's television is thought to have to be particularly colourful and fast-paced (try watching it for yourself – it's hard work!). This sensory bombardment is echoed in life in general, where the sights and sounds of modern life can be absolutely overwhelming. Music is pumped out everywhere. It is the ever-

---

* Rideout V, Hamel E. *The Media Family: Electronic Media in The Lives of Infants, Toddlers, Pre-schoolers and Their Parents*. Menlo Park, CA: Kaiser Family Foundation; 2006. Available at www.kff.org/entmedia/upload/7500.pdf (last accessed 28 February 2007). This study is one of many, providing, between them, a percentage range for children who have television in their bedrooms of 33% for 3-year-olds, 55% or more for children entering school, rising to 70% for all children. Figures are remarkably similar for the UK and the USA.

present backdrop to our lives – it is there when you shop, when you go for a cup of coffee or a meal, when you visit your hairdresser or when you go to the supermarket. Video screens are everywhere, even in post offices and banks. In many city shopping centres, large viewing screens have been erected that broadcast a continuous stream of news and sports events. In others, piped music blares out over the shoppers.

All of these things combine to produce sensory over-stimulation, as well as acting as an impediment to social interaction. Speech and language therapists are finding that more and more children have delayed speech and language skills, and have advised parents to switch off the television and talk to their children instead. Background noise militates against children developing listening skills, as well as speech and language skills, and adds to the 'sensory bombardment' mentioned earlier. One of the ways in which some children cope with this is to cut off from it – in other words, *they learn not to pay attention*. Other children might become so used to the sensory overload that they seek to create the same level of stimulation that they are used to. In other words, in a less stimulating environment (such as school) *they will behave in a way that increases stimulation in themselves and others*.

Are adults immune from this process? Experience would suggest that they are not. In the world of television it has become widely accepted that the pace is now faster, with more intercutting, rapid cuts, edits, zooming, panning and lots of action. According to one of the interviewees in Robert Kubey's book, *Creating Television*, programme makers feel that 15 minutes is about the concentration limit for today's audience. One interviewee describes the viewing public as having an attention span 'equivalent to that of a gnat.'[2]

The changes in the way in which television programmes are made echo the myriad developments that surround us in our day-to-day lives, all of which require us to be able to make rapid shifts of attention and to multi-task. For example, in October 2005, T-Mobile ran a double-page spread in the *Observer* magazine advertising their new *web'n'walk service* with the headline 'Keep movin'.' The subheading tells us: 'Every day we are faced with more choice and less time. Imagine what you could achieve if you could access the real Internet while on the move.' The pictures show a young woman using her phone in various on-the-move situations – while walking along, while standing in what looks like a park, and while with her child outside a flower shop. The text reminds us how modern life requires us to do more and more multi-tasking and how we need to 'stay ahead of the game.' Just reading it makes me feel exhausted.

Whose attention problem is it?

Television, Play Barns and games consoles are just a few of the things that stop us attending to our children. This is part of a general tendency for parents not to attend to children – that is, unless they have to. Children need our attention and rely on this to give them feedback about their behaviour. Parents who ignore their children's routine attention-seeking behaviours until they rise to such a level that they can no longer be ignored are falling into the trap of teaching their children that if they just keep up the attention seeking they will get what they want in the end. The parents end up paying attention only to bad behaviours, and in doing so they teach their children a powerful lesson – be badly behaved in order to get what you want.

The restaurant scene

I recently sat at the next restaurant table to a large family who were celebrating the birthday of one of the adults. There were two toddlers and one boy aged about eight or nine. The adults ate and drank and, when the main course was over, talked among themselves. The boy behaved exceptionally well. In fact, this is what drew my attention to him. After a considerable length of time he started to get bored and wandered over to a couple of games machines in the corner of the room. He spent about 10 minutes looking at the displays and playing with the buttons. During all this time not a single adult spoke to him. He returned to the table as the dessert arrived, sat down and started to eat. Halfway through, he started trying to attract his mother's attention, but she carried on talking to someone else. Eventually, as the volume of his voice increased, she turned to him and said crossly 'What?' He replied, through a mouthful of dessert, 'My filling's come out.' His mother handed him a napkin and told him to spit it out and not to make a fuss. The adults carried on talking. After a little while, the boy got down from the table and again went to look at the games machines. He returned to sit next to his mother and tried to get her attention, at first by whispering, 'Mum, can I have some money to play on the machine?' Only after several failed attempts to get his mother's attention did he become more insistent. She responded crossly, asking him what he wanted. He again asked for some money to play on the games machine and she told him to 'Behave.' He asked once more and got the same response. He started to whine and ask why he couldn't have some money. She gave him some. The scene was repeated 5 minutes or so later, after he had spent the money. By this time, the mother was well and truly fed up. She ignored him for as long as she could and then started complaining to the adults around her about his behaviour and how naughty he was.

I have chosen this example because of its ordinariness. It's not an example of terrible behaviour or terrible parenting – what is striking about this scene is that it is so common. The boy received no 'positive attention' from any of the adults and none from the adult who mattered most – his mother. No one told him how nicely he was eating or how well-mannered he was, or commented on his good behaviour at the table. His mother did not attend to him at all, except in response to those behaviours she considered 'naughty.' Had there been more attending to the good behaviours, he would probably not have left the table at all. As it was, no one noticed either when he got down from the table or when he came back. His behaviour gradually deteriorated as he became more bored and continued to receive no positive attention. He then got what he wanted (money for the games machine) by coercion. By the time his mother started to use the word 'naughty' in relation to him, it had become a self-fulfilling prophecy. He started to sulk and behave uncooperatively. His mother complained to the other diners about his misbehaviour. They all got up to leave. The man whom I assumed to be his father told him that he was not bringing him again – next time he would have to stay at home.

I felt very sad about the scene I had witnessed, because it could have been so different. Here was a very well-behaved child whose parents had shaped up his behaviour to be naughty. They had done this not by being 'bad' parents, but simply by not attending to him and by only responding to behaviours that were negative. When they did respond to what they perceived as naughtiness, their responses were disproportionate, pushing the boy towards bad behaviour. And what is the moral of this story? There are a couple – positive parenting is everything, and negative parenting gets you bad behaviour (and, I suppose, a third – never sit next to a child psychologist when you're in a restaurant with your children!).

What can we conclude so far about the way we parent our children today? We have a hands-off approach. We teach our children not to bother to expect to engage with us at the level of play, or to be attended to in positive ways. We teach them to expect high levels of sensory stimuli, and that their consequent accumulation of tension and irritability also gets them attention (there is no 'right' and 'wrong' kind of attention, as all parents come to realise, sometimes too late – in the child's world, *all* attention from your parents is good). We also teach our children how to be coercive.

Family problems: 'I can't understand it, they've got everything'

Parents do not have very much time together nowadays, and there is correspondingly much less family time than our own parents and grandparents will have had. Increased mobility and the lack of traditional extended family also means that most parents receive no additional support with caring for their children – it's down to them to do everything. For them, there is no time off being a parent. Most twenty-first-century families do not even sit down to eat together. When I have agreed with families whom I meet in my own clinical practice that they might like to do this, it has often proved surprisingly difficult for them, so ingrained has the habit become of each family member doing their own thing. Quite a few families have had to borrow a dining table before they could even think about the meal!

BOX 5.1 Tracey's story

Tracey is a shift worker. She leaves the house before the children get up for school. Her eldest daughter, Danielle (aged 16), has the job of getting her two younger siblings up and off to school. The problem is that they don't go. Lee (aged 14) has not gone to school for over a year now. Instead, he hangs around with a local gang and gets into trouble. He has started drinking and smoking cannabis, and was recently involved in a violent assault on another young person, for which he is due to appear in court. Lee already has a criminal record, and Tracey worries that this time he will be sent to prison. Lee's younger sister, Katie (aged 10), sometimes manages to get to school but is rarely there before 11.00am. Lately, she has been refusing to go. She was recently suspended from school for fighting after another girl called her a 'scutter.'

Other parents whom I meet are simply not at home for long enough to parent their children. Some are not there when their children go to school and are still not around when they get home, like Tracey (*see* Box 5.1).

Tracey had always had problems coping with the children. When I met her she had been a lone parent for over 10 years. Her husband was still around, but she had mixed feelings about involving him in the children's lives because of his violence towards her over the years. She felt bad that the children seemed to be going down the same road as him, always fighting. Her eldest son had been living with her parents for the past 5 years because she couldn't control him. She told me he still came back now and again and demanded money and cigarettes, which she gave to him because, as she puts it, 'she will do anything nowadays for a quiet life.' (On a couple of occasions he had smashed doors and windows because she had tried to say 'no' to him.) He had been diagnosed with ADHD and is on medication so, as she told me, 'He can't really help it – it's the way he is.' She had started to worry that there might be something wrong with Lee, too.

Tracey was working extra shifts to pay off the fines she had received for not sending the children to school, so she wasn't there in the evenings either. The children were used to getting their own food and sorting themselves out. Tracey confessed that sometimes she was glad not to be at home much because of all the fighting and arguing. I could really sympathise with her when she told me this. She felt so helpless and family life was so desperate. She made herself feel better about working by reminding herself that the children tell her that they prefer her to work so that they can have things – if she didn't work, she said, 'they wouldn't be able to have anything.'

Tracey, like many parents, does not connect her behaviour with that of her children. She is not there to supervise them, feed them, get them to school, settle them into any kind of routine or help them with their homework. Her explanation for their getting into trouble, fighting and not going to school is that there is 'something wrong' with them. This has been confirmed to her by the fact that her oldest son has been given a diagnosis of ADHD. Tracey admits that his behaviour has got worse, not better, since his diagnosis and treatment with Ritalin. I suspect that his behaviour is worse because he is now seen as having a disability that means he is not responsible for his behaviour. As Tracey says, 'He can't help it – it's his ADHD.'

This is a true story – except that Tracey's name and those of her children, along with a couple of other identifying features, have been changed. I meet many mums like Tracey in my working life, who have been so oppressed by domestic violence, depression or anxiety, poverty and debt (in a variety of combinations) that they feel helpless in the face of all their problems. Sometimes these mums have their own mental health problems arising from their own experiences of growing up. For Tracey, memories of being sexually abused as a child would sometimes overwhelm her. She is just one of many mums whom I see who try very hard to cope with family life but have just become defeated by it.

What's happened to family life?

What *do* families do together nowadays? The answer, generally, is very little. One of the few family activities (apart from watching television) seems to be shopping. Unfortunately, this is another experience that can be highly aversive for young children. Go to your local supermarket and I can guarantee that if you are there for long enough you will witness some ear-piercing temper tantrums (from the children, that is), and parents who quickly start to look as if they've lost the will to live. Weekends nowadays seem to be characterised mainly by family outings to 'the shops.' I wonder who really enjoys these trips.

Work has changed, too. Parents work such long hours that they arrive home exhausted. There is no longer any 'slack' in anybody's system. *When Mum and Dad get home, all they want to do is switch off. The last thing they feel like doing is 'switching on' to parenting.*

All of this might sound as if as parents we just can't be bothered with our children. This is just not true. Parents typically work hard for their children and place a very high value on their children's happiness. The unfortunate aspect of this is the all-pervasive message of capitalism – 'things' make for a better life. Being a good parent has become equated with getting 'things' for our children. The truth is that having too many things is a problem for them, not an advantage. Children do not need these things. They need us.

If we start to think about this, we might have to question whether we need them as well.

The real problems of childhood and family life

What are the real problems for families nowadays? They include the following:

- lack of family life (how many hours do parents spend with children?)
- parents who are absent from their children (not just physically but also emotionally)
- parents who do not attend to their children when they are with them
- parents who have unrealistic expectations of their children
- parents who have got the message (somehow) that what they do doesn't matter
- parents who feel that they cannot trust their own judgement any more, and look to 'experts' to tell them what to do.

By the way, this is not a criticism of parents who work – I'm one of those myself! In fact, some of the worst parenting I have ever witnessed has been in households where both parents are physically present. It is the *quality* of parenting that is important. Every interaction that parents have with their child is hugely important and is an opportunity, as each interaction communicates to your child that they are loved and valued, simply because you respond to them – it's that simple.

What's the problem with education?

In the UK, the National Curriculum puts pressure on teachers to ensure that children learn certain things at specific stages of their education and that this is then demonstrated through national standardised tests. Primary schoolchildren are routinely given homework. (I am fortunate enough to have started school during the 1960s, when there was no expectation that 5-year-olds would do 'proper' work. In those days 'discovery learning' was the fashion, and it was believed that children should be able to move freely around the classroom.* Thankfully, homework was something I didn't know about until I was at secondary school.)

Homework causes huge problems for children and parents. Ask any family therapist what causes family rows, and this one will be near the top of the list (along with 'the bedroom'). Begun far too early, homework is one of the many things that make learning an aversive experience for children. Parents complain to me that their children won't or can't seem to settle and organise themselves to do their homework. Their homes become a battleground as soon as they try to 'make' their child do the latest assignment.

What many parents do not realise is that, just as with play (and other skills), homework skills also need to be taught. Those who parent with a fair degree of structure and routine will deny passing these skills on to their children, but they do pass them on – they just don't notice that they are doing so.

The fact that children struggle to settle to doing their homework, or to do it properly, is not evidence of any kind of brain disorder – it is evidence that they are ordinary children. Just like us, children get tired and fed up and need time to relax when they come home after a busy day. They also have many much more interesting things that they would rather be doing, and homework can seem like an unattractive option. Most importantly, though, a child who has not been taught self-discipline, organisation skills and how-to-do-their-homework skills will inevitably struggle with this task, especially if they are left to their own devices.

On learning . . .

In recent years there has been a considerable focus on children's learning and on *how* they learn. This has been reflected in changes in teaching methodology. Within the last couple of generations the idea of early learning has been emphasised – at its extreme, through methods such as 'hothousing.'† This, along with other similar approaches, is based on the idea that we should try to educate our children as early as possible. Give

---

* The Plowden Report of 1966 was a review of primary education in England. It emphasised the need to consider children as individuals who learn through their own actions, facilitated by teachers. Plowden regarded one of the main educational tasks at primary level to be the strengthening of children's intrinsic interest in learning. Key themes in the report were individual learning, flexibility of the curriculum, the importance of play and the environment, and learning by discovery. Evaluation of learning was important but, the report cautioned, it should not be assumed 'that only what is measurable is valuable.'

† 'Hothousing' is a term used to describe the process of engaging young children in programmes of activity designed to accelerate their learning. One such example is 'Baby Einstein' in the USA, which consists of an 'educational' video and accompanying materials designed to be used with babies as young as 1 month old.

them a head start and they will learn better. So-called 'educational toys' also play on parents' eagerness to get their baby learning as soon as possible.

What parents, and sometimes teachers, fail to appreciate is that *you can't stop children learning*. They are learning every minute of the day, from the moment they get up until they go to sleep at night. This can be a real problem for adults, who have to be constantly aware that if there are children around they will be learning from us, whether we want them to or not! Children do not have to be 'made' to learn. In fact, the paradox is that when we try to do this, it usually doesn't work. However, as John Holt points out in his seminal book, *How Children Fail*,[3] parents fear allowing their children to learn and develop without coercion. We want our children to do better and to be better than us. We entrust this job of making our children 'better' to the teacher.

As early as 1964, Holt, himself an experienced teacher, began to explore what made an effective school. He concluded that it was what happened when children 'failed' that distinguished an effective school from an ineffective one. If students did not learn, the effective schools did not blame the student, their family, their neighbourhood, their attitudes or their nervous system. Instead, when they realised that they were doing something that didn't work they stopped doing it and tried something else.

This is good, old-fashioned teaching talking. It is a sensible and child-centred solution that teachers would probably not have the opportunity to consider today, when every step of the National Curriculum has been standardised and the teacher's job has become more about 'delivery' than about teaching.

This brings us to the central dilemma of education. What is it for anyway? Is it for life or for employment? If you have rushed past this question (because it seems naive or stupid), it might be a good idea to return to it for a moment or two. It has not always seemed such a self-evident truth.

In the past, working-class children were educated for work, with the routines of school mimicking those of the factories and farms. Rich parents sent their children to public school,* where they received a different type of education – one that did not seek to educate them for work but to take up their rightful place in society (at the top, of course). Over time, the idea of education *for work alone* has taken root and grown to such an extent that this has now become its sole reason for being. There are few challenges to the 'tick-box' approach to education, in which children are coached to pass what they need to pass in order to get the required grade in their exams. Thus we have the situation where, when they take their standardised tests, children appear to have learned things that in reality they haven't. This process is starting earlier and earlier, as evidenced by the fact that careers information for primary schoolchildren has recently been hailed as a good idea. At the same time, more and more children are 'failing' – they fail to reach high enough standards in basic skills, and they fail to learn how to learn. Of course, many of these children do not appear in the statistics because they are not in school at all.

Holt provides a sound argument for reviewing how we educate our children,

---

* Public school in the UK means exactly the opposite of what it means in the USA. These are fee-paying, exclusive schools.

telling readers that 'we made a terrible mistake when (with the best of intentions) we separated children from adults and learning from the rest of life, and one of our most urgent tasks is to take down the barriers and let them come back together.'

What does it all mean?

This chapter has presented a brief summary of some of the key ingredients of modern life that make some of us suspicious that it might indeed be 'rubbish.' The pace of life is now so fast that few of us take lunch breaks any more (few of us have anywhere to eat lunch, anyway), we have little time to spend with our partners and children, and the imperative seems to be to keep moving, to keep busy and to stay 'ahead of the game', to quote the T-Mobile advert. Leisure time doesn't exist anymore. If you have the odd hour or two to spare, the idea is that you should get to the gym, quickly. Weekends are generally given over to shopping and 'DIY' as a result of the ever increasing imperative to spend and improve. (When will we be good enough?) Wherever we go we are bombarded with sound and images – the soundtrack to modern life can seem inescapable. Although most of us are materially better off, the quality of our lives has not necessarily travelled in the same direction. The subjective feeling of many is that it has gone down.

The impact of these changes on our children has been enormous. There is not a single area of their lives that has not been invaded by the changes, and they are exacerbated by changes in family life, reduced opportunities for play and exploration, and altered expectations of their behaviour both at school and in the community. Could any of these things be influencing the way that they are behaving? Could it be us? Decide for yourself.

CHAPTER 6

The lost boys

What are little boys made of? What are little boys made of?
Snips and snails and puppy dogs' tails – that's what little boys are made of!

There used to be an expectation that boys would be naughty. This was a 'truth' echoed in children's literature throughout the world. A great many stories focused on the scrapes and adventures had by naughty boys, who usually survived (by the skin of their teeth) by using their wits, from the 'Just William' stories in the UK to 'Tom Sawyer' in the USA. Every culture seems to have its own 'naughty boy' stories that both children and adults love to read. It is interesting, then, that modern society no longer seems to accept naughtiness, whether in boys or girls. Naughty behaviour is seen nowadays as evidence that there is 'something wrong' with the child. Even the word itself is in the process of becoming defunct. Where children were once 'naughty', they are now 'conduct disordered' or have 'oppositional defiant disorder' or, the latest, 'ADHD.'

Nowadays, it seems, boys are big problems. They are more likely to be excluded from school, more likely to be brought to a mental health clinic, twice as likely as girls to be diagnosed as having a 'mental disorder', more likely to get into trouble with the police, and more likely to commit an offence and find themselves being given a custodial sentence.

Studies tell us time and time again that boys are much more likely than girls to be given a diagnosis of ADHD. Overall, the odds of boys attracting a diagnosis of 'hyperkinetic disorder' are *six times* those for girls, and they are three to four times more likely to be prescribed Ritalin.[1] Why is this? If ADHD is a neurobiochemical disorder, why does it seem to occur mostly in males? What is wrong with boys?

Some people think that there is nothing really wrong with boys at all. Their explanation is that social and cultural changes have impacted on how boys' behaviour is viewed, making us regard their behaviour as 'abnormal.' It is argued that the kinds of skills and characteristics that are most valued nowadays are those traditionally thought of as 'female' ones. These new values are most evident at school, where what was previously thought of as acceptable 'boy behaviour' is now considered problematic and unacceptable.[2] There is no longer room for the kind of physical exuberance, boisterousness and competitiveness that our grandparents might have had in mind when they used the phrase 'Boys will be boys.'

Other ideas about 'problem' boy behaviour focus on the ways in which neighbourhoods and families have changed in response to the escalating 'Western' capitalist ethos. Still others point to the 'innate' differences between males and females, and how these fit with the demands of modern life. All of these ideas have some contribution to make to our understanding of why it is that boys' behaviour seems to have become such a problem for us. Ironically, it's an area where the biological theorists don't seem to have too much to say. Biological theories do not seem to be able to explain this sex-linked epidemic. What can psychosocial theories offer?

Perhaps it's best to start at the beginning.

Evolutionary psychology and ADHD

Evolutionists believe that the human mind has been shaped over the course of evolution by the process of natural selection. Just like other animals, humans have adapted in specific ways to their environments and the challenges posed by them. For example, the helplessness of human infants was resolved by the evolution of the human attachment system, which ensures that infants stay close to their mothers and mothers remain responsive and protective of the infant.[3]

Some evolutionary theorists suggest that in the distant past, when we lived in 'hunter–gatherer societies', some of the characteristics that we now include under the ADHD umbrella might have been helpful – not just for the individual, but for the community. It would have been advantageous for the social group to have included those who were good at rapidly scanning the environment and acting quickly. The features of 'ADHD' – impulsiveness, hyperactivity and transient concentration – would have been advantageous to the hunter in a potentially hostile environment. In these circumstances, they would need to be hyper-vigilant and ready to respond, constantly scanning the environment for potential threats. Over time, as environments changed and became more settled and organised, these qualities would no longer have been needed. Different sets of skills and attributes would be required, such as self-control and problem-solving capabilities.

The *hunter versus farmer* theory of ADHD was first proposed by Thom Hartmann,[4] who came up with what he thought of as an 'antidote' to the often cited description of ADHD as being the product of a 'damaged brain.' He first used the idea of hunters and farmers as a metaphor, but came to regard it as 'as good a theory as anyone has.' Hartmann's proposal is that the cluster of behaviours which we call ADHD consisted at one time of *adaptive* behaviours. This theory suggests that 'hunter' attributes gave way to those of the 'farmer' as societies developed from being nomadic hunter-gatherers (where the gatherers tended to be women) to more permanent settlements. The *hyper-focus* that had been a necessary and positive attribute for the successful hunter was no longer needed. Thus it is males, rather than females, who tend to have the attributes that make them *rapid responders* – hence far more boys than girls are diagnosed with ADHD. Human evolution has simply failed to keep pace with the changing world. Conversely, critics of the evolutionary hypothesis argue that ADHD characteristics are not adaptive and would render the child more, not less, at risk in a hostile world.[5]

Whatever one's views as to whether ADHD-type behaviour could be adaptive or not, it is only relatively recently in our history that we have been required to be self-regulating, problem-solving, forward-planning individuals. In the past, when children were required to behave in this way – for example, being expected to sit still and behave in church – there would have been rigid social expectations and sanctions to ensure compliance. This is not so in today's world. Today's adults expect children to be *wholly* self-regulating in a society that has become almost devoid of social structure of any kind.

At the end of the day, let's face it, we simply don't know what kind of behaviours our ancestors would or would not have found useful – we can only guess. What the evolutionary approach does, however, at the very least, is to emphasise that what are considered positive attributes in one situation are not considered to be so in a different set of circumstances.

Sex-differentiated behaviour

Evolutionary theory is complex and extensive, and doesn't only offer hunter-farmer explanations of why it is that boys are more likely to attract diagnoses such as ADHD. One of the most fundamental things that it does is to make predictions of sex-differentiated actions that encompass a wide range of behaviours. For example, it suggests that males will pursue a more high-risk strategy than females, and will be more prone to risk-taking and exploratory behaviour. Males would also be expected to score higher on sensation seeking, risk taking and impulsivity, and lower on caution and fear.[6]

Evolutionary theories also predict that males would gain more from aggression and social dominance (because these attributes would increase the likelihood of mating opportunities). Females, on the other hand, would be predicted to benefit less from aggression and social dominance, and more from trust and empathy as supporting longer-term relationship opportunities.

Socialisation

Although there is some degree of debate about the extent to which innate behaviours of males and females determine behaviour, most evidence suggests that gender roles are more likely to be the product of the different socialisation processes experienced by boys and girls (*see* Box 6.1).

BOX 6.1 How we socialise children

Cross-cultural evidence suggests that, for the most part, gender is socially and culturally formed. Family, community and society at large treat male and female infants differently right from the start, and begin shaping their gender-role identities soon after birth. By the time they are 2 or 3 years of age, boys and girls are already aware of gender roles and stereotypes.

cont. overleaf

BOX 6.1 (continued)

Their 'blueprints' for male and female roles are quite fixed at 4 or 5 years of age, and they will try to behave accordingly. Throughout these early years, 'desirable' male and female characteristics will have been encouraged – a process that will go on throughout life. For example, girls will be encouraged to be aware of the feelings of others and to be nurturing. Boys will be encouraged to be physically precocious and to express, rather than suppress, anger. Once at school, gender-role construction continues, aided and abetted by other factors, such as social class and local cultures.

Changing families and boys without role models

In our present society, boys may be in almost entirely female-taught environments at school, as the vast majority of primary (grade) schoolteachers are female. In the UK, for instance, a mere 13% of primary schoolteachers are male.[7] Although research suggests that children's performance is unaffected by whether their teacher is male or female, it is not performance that is at stake for some children – who have no male role model and therefore no positive gender 'blueprint' for their lives.

A sizeable number of families today are lone-parent families – many headed up by female carers, so it is by no means unusual for boys to be growing up in a family without a father. Although this can be a positive choice for some families, it can also be fraught with difficulties for boys as they grow and develop. Whereas girls' developmental task is to be 'like' mother and to identify with her, young boys develop an identity 'other than' mother. This can become a problem if there is no significant male figure around for the boy to identify with. Being 'other than' is not an identity at all – it is a non-identity. Some boys experience a series of transient male 'father figures' who move in and out of their lives. Although some of these might be positive role models and might begin to develop close and supportive relationships with them, they eventually end up leaving. Others might be hostile, abusive and rejecting, both to the child and to his mother. These two scenarios are equally damaging in their different ways, and both end up compounding the problem. Discussions of 'male role models' in this context might muddy the waters somewhat, as they are not the same as fathers, and perhaps we should stop pretending that they are.

Fathers

In thinking about the development of children, psychologists have tended to focus almost exclusively on the role of the mother. In the past this has led to something of a mother-blaming culture in the literature, and to a scapegoating of mothers whenever things went wrong. Only recently has the role of the father begun to be recognised as being equally important. Neglectful, abusive and rejecting fathering is undoubtedly damaging to boys,[8] but so is being fatherless. Boys and girls who do not have fathers are disadvantaged on a number of fronts (not least economically), but boys seem to fare much worse as a result of the loss or absence of their fathers. For mothers alone, the task of raising adolescent boys can be difficult, as their natural push towards independence during adolescence brings with it challenging behaviour which can be dominant and controlling. Many families I have worked with have been very deeply affected by this, ending up with adolescent boys in equal-to-mother or even dominant parenting positions. Although they have struggled to obtain this position, it gives them much more autonomy than they are able to cope with developmentally. The most pathological examples of this have been the (thankfully) few women I've met who have replaced their violent ex-partners with sons who are encouraged to discipline their younger brothers using violence. Being put in an adult position like this is difficult for any child, but especially so when they are relegated to the role of 'child' if another partner for their mother appears on the scene. For these children it is a case of 'act like a child – but only when I want you to.' Perhaps one of the most important roles of the father in the family is to make sure that the male child is able to remain a child, as the adult male position is filled.

Good fathering is about having an equivalent role to the mother with regard to the bringing up of children. Two parents who support each other add meaning to the old adage 'Two heads are better than one.' However, it has been suggested that mothers' and fathers' roles are different, and specifically that fathers might play an important role in emotion regulation by being involved in the emotions of their children and helping them to process difficult emotions.[9] Children whose fathers are able to do this in a way that is helpful to their children have children who score higher on tests of 'emotional intelligence', which we'll come to later.

Running, jumping and climbing trees . . . so what do boys do nowadays?

The previous chapter discussed how the nature of children's play has changed over the last few decades. Perhaps one of the main characteristics of play today is that it has become more controlled by adults. It has also, by and large, moved from the streets and parks to 'indoors.' Children on the streets are assumed to be up to no good, especially if they're boys. Boys who meet up in car parks to skateboard or to play football or hockey are quickly moved on. Street football – which was big when I was a child – is an absolute no–no and would now doubtless lead to an Anti–Social Behaviour Order (ASBO). Teenagers who congregate with friends outside shops or in shopping precincts are often moved on 'because they're not buying anything' or 'they put the other customers off.' In fact, there are few areas where young people can meet up with their friends and engage in appropriate activities – unless they are 'designated' areas for young people, like skateboarding parks. Although some towns have reasonable leisure facilities, it costs money to use them, and priority is usually given to adults. Ironically, the children who are most in need of these facilities are also likely to be those who do not have any money with which to access them.

As already discussed, parental concerns about safety mean that today's children are unlikely to be left unsupervised outdoors to have the kind of adventures – naughty or not – that their parents and grandparents enjoyed. A great many boys therefore end up spending most of their time at home, in their bedrooms, playing on games consoles or computers. Some of them, left to their own devices, roam the streets. Unfortunately, modern society also finds the latter option unacceptable.

Demon kids

In May 2005, the Bluewater Shopping Centre in Kent became the first of its kind to ban baseball caps and 'hoodies.' The ban was supported by the Prime Minister, Tony Blair, and was adopted by supermarkets and shopping centres across the country. Bluewater was a clear reflection of the growing negative and fearful attitude towards young people, especially young males, exemplified by an increasingly authoritarian culture. In this new culture, you didn't have to commit a crime to be in trouble.

To date, hundreds of ASBOs have been served on young people in the UK, a policy that effectively criminalises them, even though they have committed no offence. LIBERTY, the civil rights organisation, has commented on the subjective nature of ASBOs, which break new ground in being solely a response to whether or not you are upsetting someone, not whether you are breaking the law.

Yarnfield, a small village in Staffordshire, became notorious when, in 2004, it became the UK's ASBO capital. A total of 11 young people who were 'causing a nuisance' around the village green were issued with ASBOs at a cost of nearly £60,000* (the cost of additional processes in this case increased the costs to over £90,000). Arguably, this money could have been better spent providing community youth workers or to support the provision of leisure facilities.

According to the Youth Justice Board (YJB), up to 40 young people per month end up being criminalised for breaking the terms of their ASBOs. Some of these youngsters end up being sent to a Young Offenders' Institution, still without having committed a criminal offence. Professor Rod Morgan, Chair of the YJB until January 2007, has spoken out about the demonisation of children and teenagers who are often behaving no differently to the way other young people have done throughout history. His open resignation letter to colleagues working in the Youth Justice field was critical of government policy and the continuing criminalisation of young people that has led to the UK locking up more children than anywhere else in Europe.

Modern cultural expectations of young people are that they are 'trouble.' More than two boys together seem to constitute a gang. Most parents have stories to tell about their own children being targeted by those in authority and treated as criminals in a way that would never be allowed if they were adults. During the same week I was witness to a small group of 12- to 14-year-olds being verbally abused and ejected from a shopping-centre lift they were sharing with me (they were committing no offence other than shopping), and my work colleague's 14-year-old son was chased by *non-uniformed* police and bundled into a car. His offence was walking into town on his own to meet his friends. Frightened and running, he was shouting out to shoppers to help

---

* The total cost of an Anti Social Behaviour Order has been calculated to be £5,350. http://www.homeoffice.gov.
  uk/rds/pdfs2/r160.pdf

him, as he assumed that he was being abducted. His worst fears were realised when he was put in a headlock and dragged into their car. At this point, he was screaming to passers-by 'Call the police!' The police explained later that they thought they had seen him throw a firework.

This is not to deny the fact that there are young people who become involved in petty crime in their neighbourhoods and create a great deal of misery and unhappiness for those who live there. Unfortunately, these young people seem to attract a lot of publicity at the expense of the majority of youngsters who are not 'troublemakers' but ordinary children. Applying the kinds of stereotypes that we do has serious repercussions for children and young people who are trying hard to grow up in a society that is, at best, ambivalent towards them. These stereotypes have the effect of focusing solely on the actions of young people, rather than on the factors that lead them to get into trouble in the first place. They act as an effective diversion away from the real issues.

Who are the real 'naughty boys'?

A large part of my current practice involves young people in the criminal justice system. These boys have a great deal in common – so much so that sometimes it's as if they've been living the same life. Usually they have committed a string of minor offences which nevertheless have a cumulative seriousness that makes prison a likely consequence for them. Sometimes it takes just one more thing to tip the balance. Often there is an escalation of criminal behaviour over time into more serious areas. When these boys come to us they are completely lacking in the kinds of experiences that most teenagers have had. They have had autonomy without experience, and adult experience without preparation or protection. For all their macho adolescent posturing, all of them seem to be developmentally much younger than they are. Invariably my team finds itself working with youngsters who have never been on a bus on their own, have never been swimming or belonged to an out-of-school club, have never been involved in any out-of-school sports activities, or had a hobby of any kind, and have never held a musical instrument or been to a library. No one has ever shown an interest in them and helped them to acquire skills and experiences that would develop them as individuals. Left entirely to their own devices in deprived neighbourhoods riddled with crime, their course through life has been predictable.

The lives of these young people are characterised by economic deprivation, neglect, instability, poor school experiences, poor attendance and long absences from school (some of them enforced). School exclusions often lead to family breakdown, sometimes resulting in the young person being placed in local authority 'care.' These youngsters either drop out of school or are permanently excluded. As young adults there is absolutely nothing they can do, as they have a poor school record and no qualifications, which are needed for even the most unskilled of jobs (for example, a job as a builder's labourer requires completion of a college course). All of the doors are closed to these youngsters.

Of course, there is no future for this group of boys who effectively have no education. This single factor they also have in common with many of their non-offending peers. Whereas in the past it was possible to find unskilled work, there are no longer jobs for young people without basic educational skills. These boys are lost. So who is finding them? People like me – mental health practitioners. We are the 'naughty-boy catchers' of the twenty-first century.

Boys in school

There have been considerable changes over time with regard to how schools operate. This is not only evident in significant policy changes, such as the ban on corporal punishment, but is also apparent in the general loosening up on regimentation and strict disciplinarian regimes. In general, schools are much nicer places to be than they were in the past – but this comes at a cost. In order for schools to be more liberal in their overall functioning, there has had to be a corresponding tightening of parameters about what is and what is not acceptable behaviour. This has resulted in some significant changes in rules and much more of a focus on self-regulation (i.e. young people being able to control their own behaviour and emotions).

Box 6.2 gives psychiatrist Sami Timimi's account of a playground observation, during which an impromptu conversation with a teacher confirmed how boys' behaviour was being redefined by changed expectations, and in this particular case, changed rules. What results is what Timimi terms 'a new set of "naughty boys."'[10]

> ### BOX 6.2 Dr Timimi's interesting observation . . .
>
> One day when I was carrying out an observation on a particular child in the playground, I was at the same time chatting to one of the teachers. She told me that a few years earlier the school had decided to change its policy on aggression and violence amongst the pupils, such that it was now less tolerant towards it. She told me that ever since they had become more intolerant of aggression amongst the pupils, the number of exclusions, including permanent exclusions, had risen dramatically (particularly amongst boys).

What Timimi discovered, of course, was that *expectations* in this particular school had changed, not the boys themselves.

This is an observation that has been made by a number of those writing on the subject of ADHD. Some of these claim that the school culture, teaching methodology, expectations of study and marking systems favour girls.[11] For example, assignments that require cooperative working and long deadlines tend to suit girls, rather than boys, and even then they tend to suit girls who are already high achievers.[12] It is argued that schools today emphasise qualities that are traditionally associated with female behaviour, such as compassion, tolerance and understanding.[13] What has been traditionally thought of as 'boy behaviour' has been pathologised and is nowadays seen as a problem to be 'treated' (suppressed, if you like) by Ritalin. However, the Ritalin doesn't work for a substantial number of boys who continue to find it difficult to sit still and pay attention. These boys continue to struggle to cope with the modern school environment, as reflected in the data recording school exclusions. Research shows that

10% of 13- to 14-year-olds are suspended from school in the UK on the grounds of unacceptable behaviour, and boys account for 80% of all excluded pupils. In the USA and Canada there is a similar picture. And the pattern continues. If they are not thrown out, some boys vote with their feet. One study in Quebec suggests that the male high-school drop-out rate is over 40%.[14] Giving these boys Ritalin clearly does nothing to help them to make more of the school experience.

Although some authors suggest that the school culture has become more 'feminised', it has also been pointed out by some commentators that the predominant culture within Western countries is one that is in effect 'masculine', and emphasises just the opposite set of attributes, such as competitiveness, aggression, dominance and individuality.[15]

I can't be the only one to have noticed that there is a mixed message here – for girls as well as for boys. In school, you must be cooperative, forward plan and defer gratification, while controlling your behaviour and emotions. However, in the wider world, the overwhelming message is one of individualism – getting what you want, when you want it, and exercising your 'right' to be happy. In the outside world it is important to 'stay ahead of the game', and in the language of international politics, to 'hit them before they hit you.' For boys, the mixed message is amplified by peer pressure, as well as by other local cultural, family and wider social factors that help to shape their understanding of what it is to be male.

For boys, it seems that there are particular benefits to be gained by a focus that is broader than the curriculum. For instance, research tells us that it is important for children to be helped to do things that enhance their self-concept and social status at school. Rejected social status, especially among boys, is related to aggression, hyperactivity, being 'off task' in the classroom, and disruptiveness.[16]

How we behave towards boys and girls affects their behaviour, whether we like it or not. We are all responsible for a significant part of children's socialisation and gender-role identity. At school, this can become a self-fulfilling prophecy – treat a child as 'naughty' and they will soon start to live up (or down) to our expectations. As in every other walk of life, we get the behaviour that we ourselves shape.

Boys and emotional intelligence

Children develop the capacity for behavioural and emotional self-control at different rates. Some children have limited abilities to self-regulate. This may be as a result of specific difficulties, such as trauma, but most often occurs as a result of a combination of temperamental factors and 'low-control' parenting (the kind of parenting that has a low level of structure and routine, without clear limits and boundaries). Self-regulation seems to be much harder for boys, who on the whole mature at a slower pace than girls. It is important therefore that the classroom ethos allows some adaptation to fit the child's maturity and temperament. Of course, this is just as much the case for girls as it is for boys. If in doubt, it seems that more structure, not less, is the best option. Those children who are good at self-control will not suffer because of it. They will do well in either kind of environment.

Boys' delayed self-regulatory abilities might also go some way towards explaining their poorer levels of emotional intelligence compared with girls. Emotional intelligence is the term used to describe the ability to understand and manage one's own emotions, to appreciate what others are thinking and feeling, and to act appropriately using these emotions. According to theorists, it is our emotional intelligence that determines our capacity to form mutually positive relationships.

Research shows that girls and boys tend to differ in their levels of emotional intelligence, with boys predictably scoring lower than girls. This pattern seems to be evident across cultures.[17,18] According to authors Kindlon and Thompson, today's society does not equip boys with 'emotional intelligence.'[19] Unfortunately, their socialisation militates against its development (for example, imbuing them with ideas like 'Boys don't cry'). Some commentators believe that the combination of poor emotional intelligence and a sense of hopelessness is resulting in a cohort of boys and young men who are in a permanent state of crisis, as they are ill equipped to cope with life.[20] The importance of emotional intelligence has been demonstrated in a number of studies, some of which suggest that boys' ability to handle emotions makes the greatest contribution to their success, regardless of a range of other circumstances. Fortunately, emotional intelligence can be taught. For this reason there is an increasing focus on emotional literacy in schools.

Tackling poor achievement at school

There is an indisputable gender gap in achievement between boys and girls. In 1988, 32% of girls achieved 5 A–C grades at GCSE level, compared with 28% of boys. By 1999, the gap had widened by 9.1%. Since this time, the achievement gap has remained more or less the same.[21] Not only do girls leave high school with better examination results, but they outnumber boys by 56% to 44% in UK universities.

The longstanding concern about boys' underachievement at school has been reflected in a number of educational initiatives designed to close the gap in achievement between girls and boys. In 2000, the Department of Education and Science commissioned a 4-year study by Homerton College, Cambridge, to look at the methods used by a small number of schools that seemed to have successfully improved boys' performance without adversely affecting girls' performance.

After six terms of analysis, the researchers noted that some of the successful schools they studied had used 'innovative tactics', such as altering their teaching styles to break up lesson time into more manageable chunks, with 5-minute breaks. Others used a strategy of picking out the boys who were most likely to fail at an early stage and providing them with extra help. Some schools had found that single-sex lessons helped, while others had brought about 'all-round improvements' by introducing a wider range of teaching styles.[22]

Bernie Whitehorn from Okehampton College in Devon has also researched male and female performance at the College as part of a concerted effort by Devon Curriculum Services to improve boys' educational performance. His initial research suggested that girls were outperforming boys on a number of indicators. He also found that there was a difference in how poor behaviour was dealt with. Whereas misbehaving girls were verbally reprimanded, boys were more likely to receive a detention, resulting in a male:female detention ratio of 4:1.[23] A difference in treatment between boys and girls was also found by the Cambridge researchers in their study. Whereas girls tended to receive more constructive help with their work, boys were more likely to be given verbal reprimands and 'put-downs.'[24]

Whitehorn also discovered that detentions were correlated with low English scores. Boys did not tend to read for pleasure and were poorer at presentation, which was often emphasised over ability. He suggested that there was a strong link between behaviour problems and literacy problems. He also made another observation: 'If pupils don't learn the way we teach, perhaps we should teach the way they learn.'

Classroom behaviour is not just linked to teaching and learning, as one US researcher discovered when he conducted a study on running. Dr Michael Wendt looked at the impact of exercise on the behaviour of children who had been diagnosed with 'ADHD.' The study involved children running. A 6-week study led to significant improvement for the children.[25] I suspect that studies like this one confirm what many teachers have known for a long time, as well as replicating an old-fashioned solution. When I was a schoolgirl, one of my teachers used to send restless and disruptive children out for a run, or to 'litter-pick' in the playground. I was sometimes one of the litter-pickers, and at the time I didn't think of this as anything other than punishment. More recently I have begun to think that it might also have been something else. I think it was also this teacher's way of acknowledging that we'd had enough and needed a break in the fresh air. After all, a common sense adage used to be that cooped up children needed exercise to enable them to cope. Some children seem to need this more than others. Why is this wrong, rather than just different?

Although classroom strategies and differences in teaching style have yielded good results in some schools, such methods are not always transferable. What appears to be emerging from research is that it does not seem possible to take a kind of 'one size fits all' approach to raising boys' achievement. Molly Warrington and Michael Younger, who conducted the Cambridge study, have commented that despite a number of good results using different classroom management techniques, 'the key elements come down to plain good teaching.'[26] However, as we saw in the previous chapter, many things can get in the way of 'plain good teaching.'

From these studies we might conclude that there are important differences in the way in which boys and girls learn and mature. We already know for certain that there are important differences in the ways in which *all* children learn. The reasons why are complex. Perhaps we don't need to know why – we just need to acknowledge the differences. After all, matching teaching to learning styles is not new. It is a core component of good teaching that teachers have known for decades. When we standardised education with the arrival of the National Curriculum, we also allowed target-driven approaches to education to begin to dominate, as measured by repeated testing and 'league tables' of schools. Has this been at the expense of allowing our teachers to do what they do best? How much of this has affected boys' coping and achievement at school?

If we were better able to accommodate boys (and girls) whose behaviour challenges us to do things differently in the classroom, might we find that they have something special to contribute? A number of authors have suggested that some of the attributes covered by the 'ADHD' diagnosis can be positive, and that children who have an 'explorer' temperament can be more creative than those who don't. One person who believes this is Michael Wendt, the initiator of the study into the effect of running on behaviour. He suggests that the 'differences' that these children bring to the classroom can be positive. According to Wendt, 'We are not challenging some of our most gifted children. Their gift is to handle a lot of activity.'

This idea is brought home to many of us who work with children who have had a previous diagnosis of 'ADHD', or who have been told that they have it currently. One of the best descriptions I have read comes from a young person himself, 14-year-old Matt Schervel, from a piece of writing he did for his school newspaper.[27]

> Schools don't like extremists who like to think and question. They are dreamers. That doesn't mean they are wrong. They just don't fit the norm, so they are labelled and damned, labelled as ADD . . . I can't think right, and for six hours of the day, I'm not me. I'm what the system would like me to be.
>
> The schools should shape our education around our idiosyncratic minds, our quaint minds, our quirky minds, our crackpot minds, our curious minds. Where would we be without eccentric people? We need them. The system should not shape our minds with dope and low doses of speed; the system should be shaped around us.

Social class, deprivation and social culture

With much of the focus being on the performance of boys at school, we mustn't forget some basic and important facts. Of the 40,000 young people who leave school with no qualifications, two-thirds are male and they are overwhelmingly working class. This suggests that social circumstances, economic disadvantage and local culture will also impact on boys' abilities to make the most of the school experience, and might have a larger part to play in determining how boys fare. It is even more important, therefore, that these boys can be helped to have successful and meaningful experiences at school. What seems to make a difference to whether they can do well (in life, as well as at school) is *what else* is paired with their economic disadvantage.

Who's afraid of the big, bad boys?

In school, as well as outside it, we seem to be engaged in a struggle to keep boys in check. What is this about? Is it connected to an idea that they are going to turn into murderous thugs? Is this the deep-seated fear that makes us feel that we need to 'police' boys' childhood? Do we believe that all boys are criminals in the making? Is our fear of boys linked to our fears about crime, and violent crime in particular, which many people believe is rising?

BOX 6.3 The truth is out there: crime and violence in the twenty-first century

The continued media preoccupation with crime belies the fact that crime is, on the whole, decreasing in the UK and in many other countries in Europe and North America. In the UK, the risk of becoming a victim of crime has fallen from 40% in 1995 to 26% in 2003–4.[28] *This is the lowest level recorded since 1981.* The Economic and Social Research Council, which reports on police statistics of reported crimes and British Crime Survey (BCS) figures, informs us that 'Since the peak in 1995, crime has fallen by 39%, with vehicle crime and burglary falling by roughly half, and violent crime falling by over a third during this period.'[29] These figures contradict what we think we know about crime.

The overwhelming majority of crime statistics relate to crimes against property (car crime, burglary, etc.).This is in keeping with crime figures for most affluent countries or communities. Where violent crime is concerned, the most likely victims are young unemployed males. If you're black or from an ethnic minority background, you have even more chance of becoming a victim. For the rest of us, we are probably most at risk from those we know or are close to – 120 women (and 30 men) are killed every year in the UK by their current or former partner (one-third of whom will be under the influence of alcohol), and 75% of rapes are committed by perpetrators who are known to their victims.

In the USA, violent crime is also on the decrease, although you would never guess it from the media reports. Many cities report significant reductions, while the US Department of Justice confirms on its website that 'Homicide rates recently declined to levels last seen in the 1960s.'[30]

Why is there a mismatch between the statistics and what people think about crime, and violent crime in particular? This has to be – at least in part – something to do with a continuing media preoccupation with violence, through news reports, 'real-life' crime programmes, police crime series and newspaper articles (and even series of articles), which give a major focus to those news items that report violent acts. These have a cumulative effect, making people believe the world is a much more unsafe place than it really is. Most recently, the hot media topic has been violence committed by young people, particularly in school. Concerns in the UK mirror those elsewhere in Europe and in North America, where attention has also shifted to violence in schools, highlighted by a small number of high-profile cases. This is accompanied by a focus on bullying and the widespread implementation of a 'zero tolerance policy' towards violence in schools.

With all this going on, you could be forgiven for missing the fact that there is now a much lower tolerance of violence within society. Contrary to what many media stories would seem to suggest, violence and aggression are not recent inventions. The world has always been a violent place. In the past, this included such things as public torture and executions as entertainment. Violence against children used to occur commonly at home, with whippings or beatings (and later 'smacking') used routinely to punish disobedient children. At school, discipline was maintained by means of corporal punishment, using the birch, cane, stick, belt or, for younger children, the slipper. Domestic violence was ignored, as an accepted part of life. Nowadays, although these things still happen, they are considered by most people to be unacceptable, and this position has been formally adopted by society through its criminal justice system.

Over time, we have grown less tolerant of violence. This change in attitude has led to a shift in public policy so far as children are concerned, resulting in their treatment increasingly resembling the adult criminal justice system. Whereas playground fights used to be routine when our parents and grandparents were at school, they are now likely to lead to police involvement and sometimes to criminal charges, which can (and do) result in children being placed in custody. A blanket policy of 'zero tolerance' in schools fails to distinguish between types of behaviours across age ranges, and operates more or less as a mandatory punishment. Such an approach would seem to be too unjust for the adult world, where mandatory punishments were abolished long ago. Ironically, given what we know about self-fulfilling prophecies, it might well be the case that criminalising children's behaviour could lead to an escalation or an increase in seriousness that would not otherwise have occurred – call someone a criminal and they just might start to live up to their name. Not surprisingly, black students tend to suffer most. In the USA, the bipartisan Working Group on Youth Violence reported to Congress in 2000 that 'zero tolerance means that black students will be pushed out of the door faster.'[31] There is every reason to believe that this will apply across countries – after all, racism has no frontiers.

It is important to acknowledge how far we have changed in our attitudes towards violence. But therein lies the problem. As all good psychologists know, attitude does not predict behaviour – people will always say one thing and do another. The adult world is one in which adults have the power, and they can (and do) use violence when it suits them. So we have a situation in which adults can be openly violent and abusive while sometimes over-punishing children for playground aggression. Why do we do this? Perhaps we don't want them to be like us.

Violence is the prerogative of those who have power. In our culture this still means men, whether we're comfortable with this notion or not. When men commit acts of violence, we hardly notice. With women it's different, and with children it's different again. The worst legal sanctions are saved up for them. Having upset the natural (male) order of things, social explanations abandon reason and call instead upon 'evil.'

Boys and mental health problems

By now I'm sure you will not be surprised to learn that boys tend to have more of what are called 'mental disorders' than girls. The survey entitled *Mental Health of Children 2004* found that among 5- to 10-year-olds, boys were *twice as likely* to have a 'mental disorder' as girls. Furthermore, nearly 72% of children with 'multiple disorders' (more than one diagnosis) were boys.[32] Are studies such as this one really picking up 'mental disorders' when they screen these youngsters? Or are they merely re-labelling those aspects of their lives that map on to their psychosocial disadvantages? If you've read this far, you can probably guess what my answer would be.

The Mental Health of Children 2004 survey found that the odds of boys having a hyperkinetic disorder were six times higher than those for girls. This survey also found that, apart from being predominantly boys, 'almost all were white' (97%). In addition, 71% had officially recognised special educational needs and 15% refused to attend school. These children were more likely to be absent from school for long periods, and were also more likely to have changed schools (35%).

These data confirm that the 'ADHD boys' have tremendous problems at school that go much further than not sitting still and paying attention. It is difficult to get a child's special needs officially recognised (a fact that any readers who have tried this will know well). My clinical experience is that many children with special educational needs do not receive this recognition, especially those who change schools, who are absent from school for long periods or who do not attend (note that these are also characteristics of the 'ADHD' group). I suggest that the 'real' special needs figure is likely to be considerably higher. Furthermore, most teachers would tell you that at least some classroom behaviour is the result of children not coping with the educational content of the curriculum. Children who can't cope with their work often behave in ways that enable them not to do it – they are disruptive, distracting, cheeky, non-compliant and controlling. And of course there is nothing like a fight to get you taken out of the classroom.

BOX 6.4 Jon's story

Jon was referred to our programme, which provides specialist, supported, foster-care placements for young people as an alternative to custody. He was in a special education provision for children with emotional and behavioural difficulties (a so-called EBD school). His latest offence was a supposedly unprovoked attack on another young person at school (not the first). Jon, aged 15, had the reading age of a 5-year-old and, since most lessons involved reading and writing, he would refuse to do the work. When pressed, he became abusive and created havoc in the classroom. My assessment showed that he was able enough and there appeared to be no tangible reason that would prevent him from reading and writing. One of my ideas was that he had experienced very little education, especially during the early (foundation) years, when there were many family problems and when he had to spend a lot of time in hospital, owing to a medical condition: as a result of missing out on the basics, learning had become an aversive experience for him. He had therefore developed a repertoire of behaviours to distract and disrupt others and ensure his exclusion from lessons.

The philosophy in our programme is to place children in mainstream rather than 'special' schools wherever possible, so Jon started school near his foster carers, initially on a part–time timetable and with members of our team offering classroom support. He struggled with most of his lessons and refused point-blank to read aloud, as he was ashamed of his poor skills. Jon worked up to a full–time timetable, but it took a long time for him to manage without the classroom support. His foster carers worked hard to support his learning at home, and did a lot of reading with him. Six months into his placement he read aloud in the classroom for the first time. Jon completed his programme with us over a year ago and was placed back in the community with his Aunt for the remainder of his supervision order. He has continued to attend school but his school has found it hard to access the support that he needs. For most young people like Jon such support is simply not there. Services are so stretched that they are unable to offer help to all but the absolute neediest or those in crisis. Whilst Jon's situation made him extremely vulnerable, it is depressing to have to acknowledge that some children are in even more desperate circumstances. Although he has made some important changes, Jon remains in a 'high-risk' situation, in which every day he manages to stay out of trouble is a bonus.

Those of us who work with children already know that poor school attendance, school refusal and school changes are often indicative of difficult, sometimes chaotic, home circumstances. They are some of the first things that should alert us to the fact that children like Jon are probably having to live with circumstances that are less than ideal.

This is confirmed by the research data, which also show that almost half of the 'hyperactivity' sample (47%) had experienced two or more stressful life events, with almost the same number (49%) having experienced the separation of their parents (more reasons for having difficulty concentrating in class, perhaps). But it is when we read some of the characteristics of the families that we really start to build up a picture of these children.

'ADHD families'

The Mental Health of Children study reports that 43% of the children with a 'hyperactivity' label have parents with an 'emotional disorder', and 36% of them are living in families classified as having 'unhealthy functioning.' The families of these boys are also more likely to be in major financial crisis, and the parents themselves are likely to have experienced problems with the police. More of the parents are likely to be suffering a serious mental illness. These figures suggest to me that children who are labelled as 'hyperactive' or 'ADHD' are likely to be living in families where the parents themselves are struggling to cope. It is not surprising, therefore, that their children are doing the same. The figures suggest that this group of parents experiences the kind of problems that have a significant impact on their children's emotional well-being. They do not indicate how long the children have had to live with these difficulties, but for some at least the situation is likely to be chronic. We know that such circumstances lead to stress, and that some of these children will be suffering from chronic stress, which impacts significantly on their ability to concentrate, to remain focused and to learn.

You might reasonably ask yourself where the logic is in ignoring all of these factors and focusing instead on 'attention.' And where is the evidence that these children – the vast majority of whom are boys – need to be drugged because they cannot benefit from other kinds of help? You might find yourself asking, as I do, why at the very least some of these children can't be supported in developing the kind of self-regulatory skills that they need. If ever a group of children couldn't be less in need of a pharmacological solution, surely this is it.

What can we conclude about boys?

Gender roles are still based on complementarity (i.e. men are strong, women are weak, men are dominant, women are submissive, men are logical, women are intuitive). It might be said that early socialisation of boys encourages them to be 'naughty' and encourages girls to be 'nice.' Having succeeded in socialising boys to be dominant, aggressive and physically active, we are then surprised when they experience problems in a world that has become much less rule-governed and structured and less able to contain these kinds of behaviours. As a result of their socialisation, boys are in greater need of explicit limits and boundaries than are girls, especially in the school situation. However, they are unlikely to receive them, because although the school culture has become more intolerant of certain behaviours, it has at the same time focused away from structured management and towards self-regulation (children controlling their own emotions and behaviour). Poor behaviour is much less likely to be managed nowadays – instead it will be dealt with by exclusion. Thus we have school systems that have more relaxed and liberal regimes but which also manage to be rigid and controlling about what is and what is not acceptable. A target-driven culture – exemplified by 'league tables' of results – contributes to this, as it means that schools have limited spare capacity for focusing on problem behaviours. It could be argued that for boys who need clear structures, limits and boundaries *because they are poor at self-regulation*, the liberalisation of the school environment has been unhelpful.

Although there have been rising levels of interest in emotional intelligence and its inclusion in the thinking around education, I can't be the only one to be disappointed that this is driven by 'performance' issues – in other words, if you can improve boys' emotional literacy, their academic performance improves. That's great. But why does the educational focus always have to be on 'performance' in order to justify doing anything? Can't we do something because it's for the good of the children in itself? Isn't it wholly justified to include on the school curriculum those things that are helpful to children's emotional well-being? Surely, if you want good 'performance', you need first to focus on these very things. Good performance is what happens when you get the other things right.

The children who are most likely to attract a diagnosis of ADHD seem to have a particular set of characteristics. They are most likely to be from disadvantaged backgrounds where family conditions are difficult, stressful and not conducive to good parenting. They are also likely to be children whose family culture and social class expectations play a considerable part in shaping their behaviour. These are aspects of children's lives that are played down – not only by the media but also by psychology textbooks. We like to think that our society is more egalitarian than it is. However, as we shall discover, there are more problems than ever.

CHAPTER 7

Why do children *really* have attentional difficulties?

Many childhood problems lead children to have difficulty in concentrating, motivating themselves and paying attention, or to display the kind of behaviours that can easily – and incorrectly – get them placed into the ADHD category. Mistakes are commonly made. Readers might be uncomfortable about this notion, but not all of those who make diagnoses in children have the right kind of knowledge to enable them to recognise some of the diverse contributions to children's problems – in other words, *they do not always understand what they are seeing.* The experience of many skilled clinicians who reassess these children is that there are often other explanations for their difficulties.

Complexity

Many interconnecting factors combine to create a certain problem, situation or event. The idea of single causality is just plain wrong. If it were right, then everyone who smokes cigarettes would die of cancer. We all know elderly smokers who remain fit and healthy despite their lifelong habit. This is because a great many things come together to determine whether or not a person will succumb to lung cancer, including their lifestyle, the state of their immune system, the number and type of cigarettes they smoke, their level of vulnerability and many other risk factors. Mental health is even more complicated. We have to rid ourselves of simplistic notions of cause and effect and appreciate instead that numerous factors combine to create the conditions that give rise to difficulties of one kind or another, including those that are sometimes labelled 'mental health' difficulties.

Attention is just one aspect of a spectrum of cognitive (thinking and other mental) processes that may be affected in various ways by distress, whether brief or prolonged ('chronic'). We need to remind ourselves that it is common to find problems of attention in all children, whether they have mental health difficulties or not. Among those who *are* in difficulty, it is almost a given that they will have some of these problems – among others. However – and this is absolutely critical – the attentional problem does not tell you what the child's underlying problem is. It does not tell you what is really going on – *it is only one of the symptoms.*

Children who have attentional difficulties

There are many reasons why children might have some difficulties with concentration, motivation or paying attention that might lead to problems in the classroom or home situation. One of the reasons is straightforward – childhood itself. Children are by their very nature distractible, impulsive creatures, some more so than others. This natural tendency in some children is exacerbated by the way we live, as we saw in Chapter 4. In general, modern life actively militates against the development of the kinds of focused-attention behaviours we complain that our children don't show. Furthermore, what used to be thought of as acceptable 'boy' behaviour is no longer tolerated – especially in school, as discussed in Chapter 6.

This doesn't mean that all complaints about children having attentional problems can be attributed to the insidious effects of modern living and the lack of room for childhood in modern life. For some children there are very real difficulties that become manifested in the kinds of behaviours that, quite rightly, worry the adults around them. Unfortunately, since the idea of ADHD has become so successfully embedded within our culture, what people tend to focus on concerning these children is their attentional difficulties (even though there may be many other things happening that should be of concern). 'Attention' becomes the problem that is uppermost in people's minds when you visit a classroom to observe a child, discuss a family with a social worker, or take a call from a paediatrician who has just seen a child in their clinic. And of course it is the question at the forefront of parents' thinking when they come to see you with their child.

Some children – and it's a fair few – really don't have the degree of difficulty that would put them in the clinical range of anything. Their parents have a number of diffuse concerns about behaviour and 'attitude.' Once you have managed to 'bottom out' these concerns, what remains is an underlying worry that their son (it is more often than not a boy) is becoming uncooperative and hard to manage, or is underachieving at school, despite having every opportunity to do well. For these parents ADHD provides an explanation for something they would otherwise struggle to understand. This group of parents have high expectations of their children, and want to do everything they can to help them to succeed. The more frustrated and disappointed the parents become, the more alienated and 'difficult' the young person will be. My experience is that both parents and children are relieved to have their concerns taken seriously and to be offered help on a number of fronts. Sometimes I have found that the minimum of 'direct' support has been necessary, once we have had the all-important initial conversation and everything is out in the open.

I am always more than happy to have 'the ADHD conversation', because some of these children are in real difficulty, and consulting a mental health professional has been the right thing to do, never mind the starting point. But the fact that there is an attentional problem – in itself – means little. It is usually part of a much broader picture. Due to the focus on attention, this particular part of the picture is all that is seen. The rest of it is ignored or relegated to the 'back burner.'

> **BOX 7.1 Chloe – the unheard story**
>
> Chloe (now aged 15) had been diagnosed with ADHD and put on medication when she was 7 years old. Her behaviours at that time were described as an inability to concentrate at school and being disruptive towards other pupils, shutting herself away in the dark, not listening to adults and being constantly active (having difficulty sleeping, etc.). She attended her local Child and Adolescent Mental Health Clinic when she was 14 years old, as her parents wanted a review of her medication. During this consultation, exploration revealed that she had been sexually abused by her grandfather since she was 7 years old.

Chloe's story (*see* Box 7.1) is an example of what can happen when professionals leap on 'attention' as the problem. This case, and the one that follows (*see* Box 7.2), have been sent to me by Wendy Jealous, a family therapist who was a colleague of mine in my clinical team in Staffordshire, and who has since taken over as team coordinator there. She has worked hard to maintain the ethos of listening to children and families and being open to all of their stories, not just the ADHD one.

> **BOX 7.2 Nathan**
>
> Nathan was an 11-year-old boy who had already been diagnosed with ADHD and put on medication when he came to the clinic. His mother described him as not listening to her and constantly being challenging and aggressive. His school described his behaviour as disruptive and rude to adults. During a family therapy session, his mother reported that he was the eldest of five children, and that she was a single mother and had an alcohol problem. Nathan therefore often took responsibility for his brothers and sisters, who constantly challenged him and refused to do what he asked. He then took the blame when things went wrong.

Wendy wrote the following words to me: 'I think both these cases demonstrate that there are meanings behind children's behaviours which are ignored when people get locked into a belief that diagnosis and medication are the answers.'*

Underlying the attention problem, there can be a whole range of difficulties – some quite complex, some not. The following are just a few that I commonly encounter (again some are complex and some are not). The list is not exhaustive – you might be able to think of more.

Reasons why children might have attentional difficulties

- A specific learning difficulty (e.g. dyslexia).
- Lack of readiness for the formal school experience (the child is just slow to mature emotionally).
- Mismatch between chronological age and emotional maturity.
- Unhappiness, sometimes even depression.

---

* Wendy Jealous, Family Therapist and Team Coordinator, Cannock Chase Locality Child and Adolescent Mental Health Services, April 2006, personal communication.

- Anxiety.
- Sensory impairment (e.g. hearing problem).
- Experiences of being bullied.
- Family problems (of any kind).
- Domestic violence.
- Experiences of trauma (e.g. abuse, neglect).
- Poor parenting (chaotic household, inconsistent, neglectful or harsh parenting style, parents who themselves model uncontrolled behaviour).
- Lack of stability in family life (family breakdown, adults coming in and out of the family, multiple house moves).
- Attachment difficulties (arising from disrupted attachment in early childhood, neglect or other childhood abuse, or repeated broken attachments).

Often children come to mental health clinics having experienced more than one of these sets of difficulties in their lives. Sometimes they have experienced several at once.

When parenting is not good enough

Although many of the above examples can, and do, occur regardless of parental intent, some of them have to do with poor parenting. This needs some explanation. The vast majority of parents, despite worries to the contrary, are 'good-enough' parents. This means that like me and millions of other parents they manage to get it mostly right, sometimes muddling through and sometimes making mistakes. The important thing is that this muddling and these mistakes are, generally speaking, not going to do our children any lasting harm. Unfortunately, however, there are some parents whose parenting is nowhere near good enough.

Although most parents genuinely want the best for their children, some, like Tracey (*see* Box 5.1), are unable to be good at parenting (without very special help). As a result, some children have the kinds of early-life experiences that impact extremely negatively on them. They respond in a completely normal way, *by adapting to these experiences*. Unfortunately, the process of adapting to pathological experiences means that children learn to behave in ways that are themselves pathological. These behaviours are not understood as defence, survival or coping strategies. Instead, they lead adults to view the *children* as 'disordered.' My clinical experience is that it is this group of children who are most likely to attract – incorrectly – a diagnosis of ADHD.

Before we go on to think more about how the outside world affects children, it might be helpful to reflect for a few minutes on how we develop in the first place.

How children develop

Child development refers to the process of growing, developing and maturing from birth to adulthood. It includes all aspects of development – physical, emotional, cognitive and social. The development of all of these processes is dependent on the interaction between the infant and the environment. The characteristics and qualities of the environment determine *how* the infant develops, from the tips of the toes to the neural pathways of the brain. By far the most important of all the environmental influences is the family, most notably the parents – the *primary caregivers.*

In short, children do not develop in isolation, independent of everything around them. We know that their development and behaviour emerge from the care they are given and the environment in which they live. They have a unique connectedness to their caregivers, upon which *every aspect* of their development hinges.

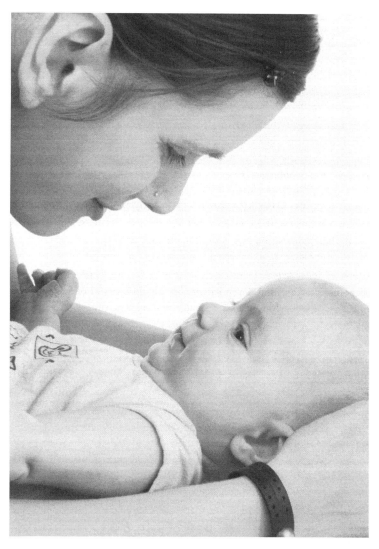

FIGURE 7.1 Attunement between mother and baby.

The importance of the primary relationship cannot be underestimated. From the start, the infant's relationship with his or her parent is unique and special. Anyone who has witnessed a new mother with her baby will recognise their intense preoccupation with each other, and their ability to exclude the rest of the world as they focus exclusively on each other.

It was this kind of observation that in 1952 led Winnicott to make his famous assertion that there is 'no such thing as a baby', and to comment that 'If you set out to describe a baby you will find you are describing *a baby and someone*. A baby cannot exist alone but is essentially part of a relationship.'[1] By this he meant that when you look at a baby, what you see is *the interaction* between mother (or father) and baby. Everything the baby does, it does in relation to them. It knows it exists, because it is responded to.

This relationship is an extraordinary one. The parents and the infant enter into an intense and intimate communication with each other through gaze, touch and sound. The parent 'tunes in' to the baby's emotional state. At this early stage, 'playing' consists of mutual gaze, facial expression, touch, body movement and vocalisation, with the parent often mimicking the baby's vocalisations in terms of pitch and intensity. These *attunement* experiences between parent and infant happen about once every 60 seconds. Thousands of them occur every day. A parent who is emotionally attuned to her baby responds to his signals and knows when to give him a rest from play, as well as when he needs her response. As the infant develops, so does the play, with parent behaviour becoming more complex in response to the child's behaviour. Such experiences are the building blocks of child development.

As a result of the quality of the parents' care, the infant develops a *secure attachment* to them. This provides a basic sense of security and trust in the world, along with the sense of being a worthy recipient of the parents' love and care. These are some of the ways in which a child comes to learn that he or she is lovable. The notion of 'fit' is critical – this sense of love and security grows out of an emotional synchronicity, and it is therefore unique between parent and child.

There are many influences on the ability of a mother and baby to respond to each other in this way. Parents' own experiences of being parented and their own attachment histories play a central role in determining what kind of parents they will be. Experiences of neglect or abuse can serve to develop parenting *blueprints* that are resistant to change.* Our own attachments as adults, as well as the sum total of our life experiences, will exert a powerful influence on how we parent our own children. Our life experiences may be further added to and amplified by other factors, all of which have an important influence on whether or not an appropriately nurturing environment can be created for mother and baby. These include the quality of the parental relationship, whether the pregnancy is unhappy, difficult or stressful, whether there is a traumatic birth, whether there is postnatal depression, and whether there are poor social conditions, parental mental illness, substance misuse or domestic violence

---

* The idea is that we all develop 'blueprints', or psychological 'working models', of our relationships, based on intense emotional experiences. The earliest one is that made by the infant as a result of their interactions with their parents. These blueprints or working models then become applied to other relationships.

– to name but a few. These things have the capacity to significantly affect our ability to become attuned to our own child's signals. Furthermore, a highly stressful home environment will continue to exert powerful influences throughout childhood.

When things go wrong

Development specialists suggest that when children receive poor care during the early years, they fail to develop secure attachments to their caregivers. Instead, they work out patterns of relating to others that reflect their learned view of the world – this world view is based on notions of dangerousness and unpredictability. These children also learn, through experience, that their needs will not be met (they might even be punished for expressing them), and that they are unworthy and unlovable (*see* Box 7.3)

BOX 7.3 Jack's story

Jack's mother had a very hard time caring for him. Her partner deserted her during her pregnancy, which had itself been quite stressful and difficult. Jack's birth left her depressed and anxious. He cried a lot. At first she tried to soothe him, but after a while she found herself getting angry. She tried lots of different things – sometimes picking him up, sometimes ignoring him. Whatever she did, it didn't seem to make any difference. He just kept on crying. He was hard to feed, too, and would just keep bringing his feeds back up. It almost felt as if he was doing it on purpose. Some days she just couldn't stand him and didn't even bother to change him. On these bad days, she didn't like handling him at all and fed him by propping up his feeding bottle on a cushion. After a while, Jack stopped crying and would just lie there in his crib. He even started crying sometimes when she picked him up. By the time he was about 3 months old, things started to get worse for Jack and his mother – her partner moved back in with them . . .

Children who are abused or neglected or who have experiences of other traumatic environments learn to survive them in particular ways. They are likely to become hypervigilant (tense, alert and over-aroused), impulsive, controlling and unpredictable. They behave in ways that can be extremely challenging. They can become very skilled at 'switching off' from things (and people) in their environment as a way of protecting themselves from further hurt – this can include switching off their own feelings. Such children also have a well-developed tendency 'not to think.' Not thinking can be a powerful defence mechanism when your past is chaotic and frightening. Unfortunately, it can also lead to problems at school and in the outside world.

Children like Jack are especially at risk of attracting psychiatric labels, one of the commonest of which is ADHD. This is because, to use one of the expressions of my good friend and colleague, Michael, they are 'spinning like tops.' Another common (but equally incorrect) diagnostic label, applied because of the way these children sometimes relate to others and seek to control their environments, is autism. Often by the time they get to see an experienced practitioner they may have collected an interesting assortment of labels. It is not unusual to find 'oppositional defiant disorder' (to explain the challenging behaviour) paired with 'ADHD' (to explain the hypervigilance, impulsivity and 'not thinking'). In older children, there may be mentions of 'obsessive-compulsive disorder', 'personality disorder' and even 'psychosis.' You might even find these children and young people on cocktails of medication (although, needless to say, their behaviour remains unchanged or becomes even worse over time).

BOX 7.4 Jack's story: what happened next

Jack was taken into care when he was 18 months old, as a result of child protection concerns. He was accommodated with experienced foster carers who understood the meaning of some of his behaviours, as they had looked after children like Jack before. Nevertheless, even as an 18-month-old, Jack had already developed some very difficult behaviours that pushed them to the limit. Despite their best efforts, the placement broke down. Jack was returned to his mother, who was to have help with developing her parenting skills. This didn't work, and Jack was once again taken into foster care, this time with new foster carers. By the time he started school, he had experienced five different foster placements. There had also been a further failed attempt to rehabilitate him to the care of his mother.

Children and young people with attachment difficulties are over-represented in mental health clinics, inpatient facilities, young offender institutions and prisons. Their difficulties often go unrecognised because those who know them and work with them focus on different aspects of their problems, without fully understanding their origins. As adults, they are unable to maintain mutually rewarding relationships. Without the proper kind of help, the cycle often begins all over again when they have children themselves.

When good parenting doesn't work . . .

Abuse and neglect are not the only things that can lead to attachment difficulties.

BOX 7.5 Steve, Alison and Josh: how one session can make a difference – so long as it's the right one

Steve and Alison came to their appointment with their 8-year-old son, Josh. They had written a long list of their concerns (two sides of A4 paper), mostly about Josh's challenging behaviour. They had tried everything, and had seen a number of different professionals over the years. Nothing had helped. Josh's teachers had suggested that he might have ADHD. The paediatrician had suggested 'conduct disorder' as well as 'oppositional defiant disorder.' A friend of the family, who had a son with autism, had brought to their attention Josh's reluctance to make eye contact and his insistence on doing things his way, raising the possibility of 'autism spectrum disorder.' Both parents felt at the end of their tether. Steve was suffering from stress

cont. opposite

> **BOX 7.5** (continued)
>
> and had started to have panic attacks at work. Alison had a longstanding depression that had started when Josh was born. She had been on antidepressants for over 7 years. Not only had Steve and Alison seen a range of different people for help with Josh, but they had also both received help intermittently for their own mental health problems. On the day they saw me, they started by saying that they were about to give up on their child.

As most clinicians would, I took a very thorough account of what had happened over the years, focusing in particular on the circumstances surrounding Alison's pregnancy and Josh's birth and early developmental history. It quickly became evident that there was a lot to talk about – we couldn't possibly get to the bottom of things in the one-hour appointment slot that had been allocated. We negotiated that the family would come back later that day after the clinic. This would enable us to piece together in detail how things had been for them, as well as help me to understand more about them as a family.

At the end of the three and a half hour assessment, I was able to share my thoughts that Josh seemed to be showing very typical signs of attachment difficulties. I explained that the stories Steve and Alison told suggested that problems had come about as a result of a chain of events and circumstances. First, an extremely traumatic birth caused significant health difficulties for both mother and baby. After the birth, Josh was incubated and his mother described being unaware of him, due to her need for strong medication. There followed almost immediately prolonged periods of serious illness and separation that militated against the development of a secure attachment. A vicious cycle resulted, whereby an unresponsive and unrewarding baby exacerbated the mother's feelings of depression and worthlessness.

Steve revealed that his father had been killed in an accident during Alison's pregnancy. He had not been able to grieve, but felt that he had to be strong for Alison and the baby. Although he told me initially that he had only recently begun to have panic attacks, these had actually begun much earlier, directly after his father's death. After Josh was born, he felt overwhelmed and not up to the task of being a father himself. Alison had been so poorly that he feared losing her as well. Part of him actually resented Josh, especially when he seemed to upset Alison so much. He, too, had found him hard to care for.

As a very young child, Josh had learned that his parents were unpredictable – they could be loving and caring, but they could also be unresponsive when they found it hard to look after him. So he never knew quite what to expect. He learned that it was necessary to control his environment and the people in it for it to be safe. He learned other strategies, too, in order to survive – all of which tended to be negative and challenging.

I told Steve and Alison a 'story' about themselves and Josh, and it was one that they responded to with tremendous relief, especially Alison. They said that no one had ever before seemed to have understood their difficulties and described them so accurately. They were puzzled that others seemed not to have known what was wrong before, despite the fact that they had had so many assessments and seen so many professionals. Why hadn't they seen the right person at the beginning?

Together we were able to discuss some of the strategies that Steve and Alison used at home to get close to their son and to explore how, gradually, they could begin to do more of what worked for them. We also discussed their general parenting approaches with Josh, some of which they now felt they would like to be different.

At the end of the meeting, they felt positive about trying some of the things that had been discussed and physically demonstrated in the clinic. Together they explored what else they felt they needed in terms of support. Interestingly, they agreed a 'package' of support that did not include 'therapy.' I agreed to remain in an overseeing role, being available as and when needed. They didn't need me.

Making sense of the problem

The relief expressed by Steve and Alison at finally feeling understood is commonly experienced by those of us working with children with complex difficulties. It is the exception to find that these difficulties have really been heard in a way that helps parents and carers to make sense of them. It needs to be acknowledged, too, that it needs a lot of the right kinds of skills to disentangle the various strands so that the essence of the problem can be determined. This includes a great deal of understanding about child development and attachment, as well as about child and family psychology. It also requires some experience and expertise in working with children and young people who have been traumatised and whose behaviour reflects this.

Unfortunately, not all doctors and other mental health practitioners who are likely to be called upon to 'make a diagnosis' in a child who looks as if they have ADHD will have the kind of background and experience that suggest they will be able to understand what they see before them.

Why is this?

The National Institute for Clinical Excellence (NICE) Guidelines (2000) stipulated that assessment for ADHD should be by either a *child psychiatrist* or a *paediatrician*.[2] They have not departed from this position. Many see this guideline as problematic, as well as surprising, since both practitioners will inevitably be viewing the child's problems through a 'medical lens.' Furthermore, while community paediatricians have little or no background training in children's mental health, child psychiatry training contains little in the way of developmental psychology. Neither of them routinely have any training in cognitive development (which includes attention and motivation) or social or behavioural psychology. However, clinical psychologists do.

In a nutshell, these are the differences.

■ Paediatricians are experts in children's health.
■ Psychiatrists are experts in mental illness.
■ Psychologists are experts in human behaviour.

Perhaps it is not surprising that psychologists' training and assessment methods lead them to different conclusions about children's behaviour. What is surprising is that NICE is explicit in making the recommended assessment medical, rather than psychological, and in doing so effectively excluding the kind of psychological overview that is needed. Although the NICE guidelines allow psychologists to 'contribute' to the assessment that is being made by the psychiatrist or the paediatrician, such a contribution is designed to add to the specific information gathering (e.g. cognitive assessment). It does nothing to change the focus of such an assessment.

The impact of trauma and what we can do about it

While some children who have experienced trauma or neglect behave in a way that suggests (to some) that they have 'ADHD', others who have clearly not experienced the same kinds of backgrounds nevertheless present in a similar way. Why might this be? The answer lies not only in the experiences that children have but in *how* they have been experienced. For some children, their behaviours have arisen from other kinds of stressful experiences – the types of sustained experiences that combine and build up over time. Or there may be specific reasons why their coping threshold is lower than that of others. Stress is a complicated thing. Box 7.6 is a reminder of how the stress cycle works.

BOX 7.6 The human stress response – 'fight or flight'

Our ancestors were well equipped to cope with threats from sabre-tooth tigers and other scary beasts that might have been lurking in the dark corners of caves, waiting to jump out at them.

At the first hint of a threat like this, their bodies would go into 'fight or flight' mode. In other words, the brain, recognising a life-threatening situation, would send a message to the pituitary and adrenal glands to release a surge of stress hormones into the bloodstream.

These hormones would act quickly to divert energy resources away from areas that are not needed in a threat situation, such as the digestive system, to those that are, such as the arms, legs and respiratory system. These areas would get the 'boost' of an increased blood supply, enabling our ancestors to either fight or run for their lives. When the threat was no longer present, the pituitary and adrenal glands would receive a signal to stop producing the stress hormones, and the system would return to normal.

As modern–day humans we have exactly the same hardware as our ancestors. The same stress feedback loop is in operation. Only now there are no sabre-toothed tigers that we have to fight or run away from. For most of us who are fortunate enough to live in situations where our lives are not under threat, the 'fight or flight' response is not particularly helpful. Modern-life stressors are likely to be the type of events or situations that require a different kind of response altogether – for example, being stuck in a traffic jam, taking an examination, or recurrent confrontations with an antagonistic neighbour or work colleague, none of which present an immediate threat to our lives. However, evolution is slow to catch up – the stress response remains the same for us in these situations as it was for our ancestors when they were confronted by the sabre-tooth tiger. Furthermore, modern life can bring recurrent daily stresses and strain for many of us, in which case continuously high levels of stress hormones may flow through the system unchecked. What was once an adaptive, life-saving response begins to have a detrimental effect, both physically and psychologically. If this process is not interrupted in some way, we know that there are increased risks of serious illnesses, such as cancer, heart disease and diabetes.

What causes stress?

Put simply, stressors are anything that places the human body or mind under sufficient pressure to initiate the stress cycle described above.

Stress can arise from a number of different sources, some of which are listed in Box 7.7.

BOX 7.7 Some sources of stress

Environmental – excessive heat, noise, pollution, over- or under-stimulation, living in a threatening environment (e.g. war, domestic violence).

Social – poverty, debt, poor housing, overcrowding, homelessness.

Emotional – fear, anger, worry, boredom, frustration, helplessness, anxiety.

Physiological – pain, thirst, hunger, medical procedures, chronic medical conditions.

Trauma – abuse, neglect, being a victim of crime or torture, accidents, battlefield experiences.

(Secondary trauma can arise from witnessing some of these events or, rarely, from hearing about them, especially if the victim is known to you.)

Some increase in arousal in the face of a challenging situation can be helpful in boosting performance or coping (for example, a certain degree of stress before a test has been shown to improve students' performance). However, too much stress is counterproductive, and chronic stress (stress that continues over time) has been shown to have negative and damaging effects. In keeping with the results of adult studies, stress researchers have reported significantly higher levels of stress in poorer children than in children from better-off families and neighbourhoods.[3] This has been shown to have an effect on cognitive (mental) processes, and is related to how children think about situations and events. The higher the stress levels, the more negative the thinking is likely to be.[4]

Stress and children

In the past, there seems to have existed a kind of mythology that children were unaffected by stress because they had the protection of *resilience*. (If this still seems like a plausible idea to you, reflect for a minute on the fact that children used to be considered less affected by physical pain, too.) The idea that all children, simply by virtue of being children, have an inbuilt resilience that enables them to endure traumas and emerge relatively unscathed just doesn't hold true. Furthermore, it does what a number of other myths about children do – it lets us off protecting them and needing to have their welfare in mind. Many studies show that children are more affected by trauma than adults, not less.

The unique position of children – that of being dependent on their caregivers for their very existence – means that they have a special vulnerability and helplessness in the face of stressful events. Furthermore, the child's level of understanding (or lack of it), which was previously thought to act as a 'protective' factor, can instead worsen the trauma and its aftermath. For example, the child whose mother is beaten by her partner fears that his mother is going to be killed. Since she is his only source of love and protection – the only one who looks after him in all the world – this means his death as well. Afterwards, the child may blame himself for not protecting his mother – even though, for a 5-year-old, this is just not possible. Young children also have a tendency to blame themselves when bad things happen, making sense of the trauma as 'punishment' for their badness. The impact of this kind of meaning-making is very significant, and its effects can be far-reaching. Furthermore, since this reasoning can take place at such an early age, it becomes an unconscious part of the way in which a child makes sense of the world, and it can be resistant to change.

How do we know that children are affected by stress?

We know when children are affected by stress because their behaviour tells us so – just like that of adults. There are also other ways in which we can confirm or disconfirm that a child may be under stress. One of these is by measuring the levels of the stress hormone, cortisol, in the body. As we have seen, when the stress cycle is set off, the body is flooded with stress hormones, one of which is cortisol. Research studies on children, some on very young infants, have been able to confirm increased levels of salivary cortisol using mouth swabs. Studies show that infants who receive consistent and responsive care produce less cortisol, while those whose quality of care is poor show elevated levels. Some studies have shown that these levels remain elevated,[5] suggesting that children with insecure attachments may suffer from chronic stress.[6] In this context it is not surprising that adopted children, who have often experienced the trauma of neglect or abuse as well as repeated broken attachments, are over-represented in ADHD diagnoses.[7]

A considerable body of literature, combining information from studies on child abuse and neglect, attachment and learning research, has now been amassed. These studies are all unanimous in their agreement about the damaging effects of chronic stress on children. Problems that are indicated include developmental delays, behavioural and emotional problems, attention and memory difficulties and hypervigilance.

Is any of this starting to sound familiar yet?

The impact of stress on the brain . . .

Research suggests that levels of stress in infancy shape the stress responses in the brain which, once sensitised, begins to affect memory, attention and emotion. The influence of stress on mental processes is significant.

. . . And on the mind

Earlier in my career I worked with a number of children who had had traumatic experiences, such as road traffic accidents. Some of these young people were suffering from traumatic stress. Part of my assessment of these children included cognitive evaluation.* I found myself fascinated by some of their results, which highlighted what seemed to me at the time to be something of an anomaly. In intelligent young people with otherwise good verbal skills, I was finding that their retrieval of information was unexpectedly poor. This did not seem to fit with the pattern of their results on other tasks, something that led me to re-score and re-analyse each one of them. After considerable reflection and discussion with colleagues (thank you, Celia), it seemed that these youngsters were 'not remembering.' This mechanism was being applied not only to information related to their accidents, but also to other information. It was at this stage of my career that I began to wonder about the role of 'not thinking' in the lives of children who had experienced trauma or who had lived traumatic lives.

Nowadays, when I meet a young person for the first or second time (often a young offender on the way to prison) and they tell me about their life, I sometimes find myself sharing with them, out loud, some of my thoughts that it might be easier for them not to think. Some of them comment on this, as one young man did, telling me 'I get angry when I think.' Although it might well have been a good coping strategy for them as young children, 'not thinking' has, for them, provided its own set of problems. Understanding this is the easy bit – changing it is not so easy.

The importance of the early years

All of this adds impetus to the importance of the 'wide-angle lens' in understanding children's problems. This means appreciating the way that everything influences everything else during the early years and what is meant by the child's environment in all its complexity. Unless we understand something of the way in which children develop amidst the tangled web of relationships that surrounds them, we risk getting a distorted picture in which some aspects are highlighted while others are masked or even obliterated.

It is interesting, and some would say encouraging, that biological psychiatry is – rather belatedly – 'discovering' developmental psychology. It is less encouraging that it seems to be seeking to repackage it as 'developmental *psychopathology*.' The

---

* Cognitive evaluation or assessment involves administering specially designed psychological tests to provide evidence of a range of cognitive abilities and function. The most well known of these is commonly known as an IQ test (although this is not how psychologists refer to it).

terminology is important, as *psychopathology* is a term used to describe abnormal mental processes, not normal ones. This is completely different from the task undertaken by developmental psychologists, who for the best part of a century have sought to understand how *all* humans develop (not just those deemed to be mentally ill), and in so doing to gain a greater understanding of how we function, not just what happens when things go wrong. There is a significantly different focus in a biologically driven, developmental *psychopathology* that looks at development in a way that still calls in biochemistry to explain children's difficulties in simplistic cause-and-effect ways. To illustrate the differences, let us consider maternal stress.

Maternal stress: different ways of looking at the same results

In 2005, it was widely reported in the popular press that stress during pregnancy was being 'passed on' to babies. Research had shown that higher levels of salivary cortisol in a group of 10–year-olds correlated with high stress scores on questionnaires completed retrospectively by their mothers about their pregnancies.[8] The researchers concluded that prenatal stress or anxiety 'predicted' mental health 'disturbances', such as depression and anxiety. Interestingly, and without any further evidence, they highlighted cortisol as *leading to* possible mental health 'disturbances', rather than arising *as a result of* disturbances in the children's lives that would have led to the increased stress levels. This is a very important difference. These are fascinating conclusions, suggesting that what you are looking for is what you get! In other words, ask a biological question and you'll get a biological answer.

Although elevated levels of cortisol indicate that the children in this particular study are suffering from stress (after all, that's why we all produce cortisol), that is just about all we can conclude from a study like this. Cortisol does not cause mental health 'disturbances', as demonstrated by the many adults who have problems with cortisol over-production, although it does lead to physical and cognitive (information-processing) disturbances. It is the *response* of a system under stress, not its cause.

The problem with (some) research

The fact is, we simply don't know enough to begin to interpret this single reported finding. The point I am trying to make is that measurement of stress itself, whether in the form of answers to a questionnaire or salivary cortisol levels, is only one indicator of what is happening in a person's life. *It is only one factor.* It is poor science indeed that seeks to elaborate from this single factor (which itself is caused by others) to conclude that there is a direct causative relationship between pre-birth stress and 'diagnosable' mental health problems (and, furthermore, that it is the *stress hormones* – almost by virtue of being passed through the placenta – and not the myriad adverse environmental and relational conditions accompanying them, that do the damage). If this kind of thinking were true, all we would have to do would be to administer an anti-cortisol pill (if there were such a thing) to a child and everything would be all right.

In order to make these kinds of cause-and-effect judgements, the researchers would have had to control for every single potential confounding variable. In ordinary English, this means they would have had to remove or make sure that no other single influence could have been responsible for the relationships between higher levels of cortisol in the children whose mothers reported having had more stress in their pregnancies. They didn't. Yet this is one of the most basic principles that would-be scientists and researchers learn – straight out of 'The Noddy Book of Research Rules', in fact.

Unfortunately, biological research tends to get reported by the media as fact. Sometimes they are aided and abetted in this by drug company press releases – they are really only repeating what they have been told. The results are framed as 'breakthrough' news items, trumpeting newly discovered relationships between one thing and another. These usually make all kinds of spurious suggestions about causation (whoops, there goes the second Noddy rule – an occurring relationship is just that, and it should never be taken as evidence that one thing has caused another, because you just don't know). You can't always blame the researchers for this, either. Any study that seems to strengthen the biological argument is taken down and used in evidence.

We are witnessing more and more reports of pseudoscientific conclusions that claim or imply causative associations. In fact, we just can't seem to get enough of them. Going through the supposed risk factors for, say, schizophrenia, would need a chapter in itself. On reading them, you might conclude that almost anything is a risk factor. For example, the myriad things that apparently increase the risk of schizophrenia range from exposure to X-rays[9] and cat ownership[10] to not being breastfed.[11] Invariably they are reported as 'evidence' of some kind of biological determinism. Simple cause-and-effect science is always attractive. It allows us to feel that we can make sense of the complex world around us. But this is seductively deceiving. It paints a grossly distorted picture of how things actually happen.

Back to stress . . .

In contrast to how they have been reported, the maternal stress studies can be interpreted as providing added support for the psychosocial understanding of development. By retrospectively highlighting maternal stress, such studies suggest that the characteristics of the family environment, exemplified by the circumstances of the mother, are critical for children's psychological well-being. Unfortunately, the researchers do not tell us what happened in the intervening years, before they measured levels of cortisol in the children at the age of 10. However, we do know that social circumstances have a habit of remaining static over time, while attachment theory also suggests that mothers who are experiencing stress (of any kind) might find it difficult to care for and bond with their children, and that ensuing attachment difficulties often result in children suffering chronic levels of stress.

If we don't simply focus on the supposed biochemistry, such information can be seen as supporting the view that it is the child's environment, rather than some notion of his or her innate biochemical characteristics, to which we need to pay attention. These environmental influences have far-reaching and long-lasting effects.

If we understand children's difficulties as emotional and behavioural responses to stressful environments and, in some cases, as indicative of their chronic stress levels, this is hardly surprising. What a pity that the researchers in this study couldn't have commented on this, rather than speculating about another supposed biochemical route to 'disorders' in adolescence, of which there is no proof whatsoever.

The importance of taking a holistic approach

Looking at development in a holistic way that also takes into account the influence of the environment on the brain is not new at all. Psychologists have been doing this since psychology developed as an independent discipline. Psychologists have always understood lifespan development in terms of the reflexive relationship between the person and the environment in which they live. Each exerts an influence on the other, and each develops in response to the other. In addition to its role as mediator, the brain both shapes and is shaped by all experience.

What *is* new (and concerning) is that what psychologists know as developmental psychology is in the process of being hijacked by biological psychiatry, which seeks to re-label these early relationships in terms of biochemistry. This is especially worrying, as those studying it will not necessarily have an understanding of the normal course of human development, in all its complexity, that predicates all psychological study. Instead of this, the understanding is to do with the biochemistry of 'abnormal' development, or mental illness. Thus within-child explanations ('there's something wrong with the child') become even more emphasised, this time with biochemical 'proof.' This is a worrying interpretation of the dynamic relationships between body, mind and environment. Of course there are relationships between the developing child and his or her brain, between the mind and the neuronal representations within the brain. But they are not one and the same, as we shall discover in the next chapter.

CHAPTER 8

A bit about the brain

In a book highlighting some of the consequences of an increasingly biological view of children's difficulties, it would be an omission not to include something about the brain, especially since so much of the pro-ADHD argument seems to be about what is, or is not, happening in the brain.

As an undergraduate psychologist I well remember grappling with the 'cognitive science' part of my curriculum – different types of attention, how we learn, how we remember, how we process information, how we store it, psycholinguistics (yes, the other stuff that Chomsky is famous for), visual processing, concept formation, and so on. These subjects make up the study of mental processes, helping to develop our understanding about how the mind works. I find myself recalling this work whenever I am trying to understand the interrelationships between mind and brain.

What is the mind?

We describe mental processes – thinking, remembering, learning, symbolic reasoning – as taking place 'in the mind.' But where is the mind? It is perhaps best, and most simply, described as the *virtual* system that corresponds to the biological system of the brain.* We can't see the mind (but then we can't see radio waves or the Internet). Neither do we know how it is related to the brain, or indeed if they are one and the same thing. The mind–brain relationship has been preoccupying philosophers and psychologists for just about as long as we've been able to theorise about it. The division between 'mind' and 'matter' was originally made by Descartes in the seventeenth century. For Descartes, consciousness (the ability to think about thinking) was the thing that confirmed that we really existed: *cogito ergo sum* ('I think, therefore I am').

Philosophical questions

The relationship between the mind and the brain is an area where debate still rages wildly, and will do so for the foreseeable future. Theories can be viewed – very broadly speaking – as variants of either one of the two main paradigms. 'Dualism' is the school

---

* This very helpful phrase is used in the following book: Giles B, editor. *The Brain and the Mind*. Rochester: Grange Books plc; 2002.

of thought that was exemplified in Western thinking by Descartes and sees the brain and mind as separate but related entities.* The often cited traditional metaphor was that of the computer, where the brain is the hardware and the mind is the 'software.' 'Monoism', on the other hand, holds that the brain and mind are one and the same thing, and that – sooner or later – all mental processes will be reduced to individual cells and neurons. (Academics out there who specialise in mind–brain philosophy will no doubt be appalled by my over-simplification of this area.)

The brain

The brain is an extremely complex organ. It makes up only a fraction of our body weight, weighing around 3–4 pounds or 1300–1500 grams. It looks like a large, spongy walnut, but its appearance belies the critical part that it plays in our lives. The human brain contains over 200 billion neurons, or brain cells, which communicate with each other by means of electrical signals. This process is made possible by the presence of different types of neurotransmitters.

Modern techniques such as computed tomography (CT) and magnetic resonance imaging (MRI) scans and functional neuro-imaging can show us the structure of the brain and enable us to 'see' which regions of the brain are involved in different activities. These techniques can highlight different regions of the brain, depending on the kind of task in which we are engaged. However, they cannot measure *activity*, only *blood flow*, which, contrary to what you might expect, does not always correspond directly to neural activity.[1] What neuro-imaging allows us to do is to 'map' the brain in terms of its particular areas of function. Although the map may vary in the detail, it is more or less the same from person to person. What functional neuro-imaging doesn't tell us (yet) is how the different parts of the brain interact.

These methods have been useful in helping to confirm long-held beliefs about phenomena such as localisation of function, plasticity, compensation, and so on.† They can help us to determine what kind of processing goes on in particular areas of the brain, but of course this type of information tells us little about subjective experience. For example, we might know where music is processed, but we learn nothing about whether the music is liked or disliked.

The importance of mental processes

The current preoccupation with neurophysiology leaves many feeling that the significance of mental processes has been underplayed. Such processes are critical

---

* Although the idea of mind–body dualism first existed in Eastern philosophy, and in the West, in the writings of Plato and Aristotle, it was René Descartes in the seventeenth century who first identified the mind with consciousness and self-awareness and distinguished it from the brain. It was Descartes who was responsible for formulating the mind–brain problem.

† *Localisation of function* refers to the way the brain is organised in distinct areas that correspond to specific functions, such as language. *Plasticity* describes the ability of the brain to adapt and reorganise in response to environmental changes and injury. *Compensation* refers to the process by which neural reorganisation can take place to enable other areas to 'take over' functions from those that have been damaged.

in determining how sensory information is processed. For example, consider seeing, which involves the visual cortex. We know which major part of the brain is responsible, as well as which other parts help, and we know the mechanics of how humans 'see', but this doesn't give us the whole picture. In order to truly 'see' – that is, to *make sense of images* – we need to be able to perform mental operations – that is, to use the skills of our mind. If someone was to ask you how many windows there are in your house, research suggests that you would form a mental image of the house and then count them. You would even be able to rotate your image, so as to have different views of your house. This is an example of how we use imagery.

Face recognition is another good example of how we use mental processes to make meaning out of what we see. Of course we need the hardware – the visual cortex – but we also need mental operations for memory and recognition. The visual cortex alone would not be enough. Seeing is therefore not just about what happens in a particular part of the brain. It is also about using experience. And depending on what our experiences are, seeing is not always believing (*see* Box 8.1).

BOX 8.1 The Muller-Lyer illusion

The Muller-Lyer illusion was created in 1889 by Franz Muller-Lyer, and is one of the most famous visual illusions. When two vertical lines are presented side by side, with 'fins' pointing either inwards or outwards, one is seen as longer than the other, even though they are in fact exactly the same length.

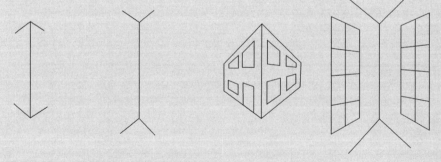

FIGURE 8.1 The Muller–Lyer illusion.

Although there are a number of hypotheses to explain why many of us are fooled by this illusion, the accepted explanation is based on what is known as the 'carpentered world.' Basically, this suggests that the illusion works on those of us who live in a three-dimensional world of straight lines, edges and corners. This affects our perception of the two lines, which are interpreted as inside or outside 'corners', as we try to make sense of them using our usual mental processes – they are adjusted according to our conceptions of depth perception. As the theory predicts, this illusion has been shown to be ineffective when shown to people from rural African communities where homes are circular and their environments lack the kind of 'carpentering' that is found in Western countries – they were not fooled by the illusion.

Neuroplasticity

The term *neuroplasticity* describes the ability of the brain to develop and adapt to changed circumstances, and it involves a range of processes. It used to be thought that adaptation and change were only possible during early childhood, while the brain was still in the process of becoming organised. However, it is now understood that neuroplasticity is a lifelong process, although different kinds of plasticity are more likely to occur at particular life stages. The brain needs to remain plastic to enable continued learning (which of course involves mental processes) and adaptation (ditto). It also needs to be able to compensate for lost or poor function, which it does by shifting brain function from one area to another. There have been some very dramatic illustrations of this (*see* Box 8.2). The brain is therefore shaped by environmental characteristics as well as by behaviour.

BOX 8.2 The 'rewired brain'

On 3 July 2006, the *New Scientist* reported on the case of Terry Wallis, who in 1984, at the age of 19 years, had been thrown from his truck during an accident. He was discovered 24 hours later, with massive brain injuries and in a coma. Wallis spent the next 19 years in a minimally conscious state, which it was thought would last for ever. In 2003, he astonished everyone by beginning to speak and regaining the ability to move and communicate. He still believed that he was 19 and that Ronald Reagan was president of the USA. He had to start getting to know his 20-year-old daughter.

Investigators at Cornell University in New York found that new pathways had developed in Wallis's brain, along with completely novel anatomical structures. These had re-established functional connections by way of compensation for the loss of neural pathways in the accident. The investigative team reported that the new pathways looked completely different from normal brain circuitry, and had grown across the back of the brain, bypassing damaged areas. Eighteen months later, as Wallis continued to improve, it was noted that some of the new pathways had now receded and others had taken over. The *New Scientist* cites Krish Sathian, a neurologist and specialist in brain rehabilitation, as commenting that 'the bounds on the possible extent of plasticity keep on shifting . . . Classical teaching would not have predicted any of these changes.'[2]

The mind–brain relationship

Whether the neuroscientists like it or not, technical developments such as imaging have had the effect of enhancing the focus on biological psychiatry by being perceived to lend it credibility. Such methodologies have been seized upon by the biological psychiatrists as finally providing the evidence they need that mental health problems are diseases caused by neurochemical imbalances. Images showing supposedly 'normal' and 'abnormal' brains are held up as the 'proof' that there is, after all, real science behind this theory. The new technologies also add to the school of thought that accepts as 'real' only what can physically be 'seen' (although what can be seen is open to interpretation, as we shall discover). As a result, there has developed a sense that it is only a matter of time before everything about the brain will be revealed and there will be no more 'mystery' of the mind. This in turn has added credence to the philosophy that what we do is determined solely by the chemistry of our brains.

Peter Sutcliffe, known as the Yorkshire Ripper, who murdered 13 women in England between 1975 and 1981 (and possibly killed many more), has left his brain 'to science', presumably so that 'science' can discover what made him a multiple murderer in the first place. How does this equate with the knowledge that we have developed about human psychology over the past 100 or so years? After all, we can argue with some degree of certainty that we already know the key ingredients of psychopathy and have done so for some time. We could also argue with absolute certainty that when we look inside someone's head we don't find their life story. The word 'murderer' will not be running through Peter Sutcliffe's brain, like Blackpool rock.* When the post-mortem analysis of his brain 'discovers' an under-developed capacity for empathy, which it presumably will do, it will be re-stating the obvious and very basic starting point of a psychological explanation (what it won't tell you, of course, is what came first). Unfortunately, explanations like this inevitably lead to assumptions about people being born with defective brains and this defect being what causes them to become murderers. The problem is twofold – it lies in the credibility awarded to biological phenomena, as well as in how they are reported and interpreted. Whenever something is described as being 'in the brain', it is undoubtedly viewed by non-scientists as being 'fixed', unalterable and scary. This is just not the case.

How the environment shapes the brain

In Chapter 7 of this book I described attachment – that is, the process by which a mutual bond develops between an infant and its parent figures through a process of intensive emotional interaction. This process is accompanied by a considerable degree of activity in the baby's brain and nervous system. Basically, the infant brain is experiencing what can only be described as a 'growth spurt.'

During the first few years of an infant's life, neuronal development of the brain occurs rapidly. At 2 or 3 years of age, the infant will have far more synaptic contacts than he or she will ever need – about twice the number found in the adult brain.[3] These are whittled down through a process known as *synaptic pruning*, which deletes weaker synapses while reinforcing stronger ones. What determines whether a synapse is weak or strong is whether or not it is used (i.e. whether it receives or transmits information). This synaptic pruning is therefore *experience dependent*.[4] In other words, the brain adapts itself to its environment.

This 'use it or lose it' process has led to hypotheses that the absence of attunement experiences, say, as a result of neglect, results in poor synaptic development. For those of you who like this kind of information, neuropsychologists have located this area

---

* For those readers who are unfamiliar with the English seaside, 'rock' is a hard, sugary sweet which has the lettering of the name of the seaside resort running through it, so that every time you break off a piece, the place name is visible.

in the right orbitofrontal cortex – the part of the brain that is thought to be essential for the processing of emotional information. This poor synaptic development, they say, explains why children with attachment difficulties have such problems managing their emotions. If they experience chronic stress, the presence of the stress hormone, cortisol, will also have a detrimental impact on the developing brain. Ordinarily, stressful experiences in the infant are mitigated by responsive, attuned responses, which help it to develop the capacity to self-regulate. (In neurophysiological language, the frontal cortex of the brain develops a greater capacity to modulate stress experiences.[5]) So the theory continues that the child who has poor attunement experiences can be doubly disadvantaged by stress, and these experiences are not only reflected in the structure of the brain, but also explain why it is that these children have the problems they do.

So far there is nothing wrong with this kind of explanation, which is in keeping with decades of learning about child development and psychological processes, as well as clinical experience (but remember that it is only a *partial* story). It describes the very basic elements of the psychological and physiological feedback loop between mother and baby, but it does so in a different language from that used by psychological therapists. This, too, isn't a problem. It only becomes one when the *biology alone* is over-emphasised and described as the *cause* of a child's behaviour (which has begun to happen more and more as the biological focus has increased). Then the explanation runs like this: *these children have problems because they have defective brains*, rather than *the psychological processes in these children develop as an adaptation to their defective experiences, some of which are reflected in structural changes in the brain, which are themselves subject to continued learning and adaptation.* The fact that mental processes are reflected in structural terms in the brain should not come as a surprise to anyone. We already know that biology is part of a complex interplay between mental processes, environment and behaviour, all of which lead to adaptations in the brain. Surely if we believe this, though, we have to challenge the notion that the 'wiring' of the brain is 'fixed.' Surely we have to believe that change in the other direction is possible.

What have we learned about attachment?

Attachment is a good area to focus on when considering these issues, as there is widespread agreement about the impact of early relationships on the developing brain. Clinical and therapeutic experience provides a rich source of information about how children with attachment difficulties progress. Unfortunately, despite its comparative sophistication, this body of knowledge seems to be undervalued in comparison with studies of physical phenomena. Presumably it lacks the 'wow' factor of 'live' images of the brain.

Although some attachment theorists consider that what happens during the early years has an indelible impact on the human brain and cannot be reversed, others do not believe this. Instead, although it seems to be universally agreed that the early years are important in 'setting the scene' for later development, they see attachment as a lifelong process, during which there can be many opportunities for change and healing.

This view is supported by clinical evidence.[6] Successful therapeutic interventions are integrative and seek to replicate earlier experiences of dysregulation, only this time with some facilitated resolution. We can only guess as to whether or not this kind of positive change 'shows' in the brain. Changes *in mind* happen when properly and skilfully facilitated. As a clinical psychologist I would see these changes in mind as the vehicles of change, in terms of both individual thinking and behaviour. If this shows at the neuronal level, that's fine. I'm sure there are some people who are keen to see it. Personally, I live with change every day and see the impact of it across all levels. Along with other psychological therapists, I do not consider that finding the physical correlates of such processes makes them any more real than they are already. Indeed, so far it seems that such a search has devalued them.

How mental health has come to be dominated by the brain

In 1990, in an act that many found supremely ironic, the US president, George W Bush, declared the last decade of the millennium to be 'The Decade of the Brain.' This focused funding and research activities on the brain and was another contributory factor in the already increasing focus on biological psychiatry.

Some of this focus has been on the search for 'hard' neurophysiological evidence, not just of 'ADHD' but also of other mental illnesses. Such a search presents us with further dilemmas, not least of which involves trying, as Grace Jackson puts it, to define and locate in the brain 'the functional equivalents of psychological distress.'[7]

Perhaps predictably, given this consideration, this search has been unsuccessful. Although it has been extensive, there is still no evidence anywhere to show that mental illnesses 'exist' in the brain. To quote Jackson again, 'more than fifty years of research have failed to confirm radiographic evidence linking any psychiatric condition to a structural defect within the brain.'[8]

This brings us on to two important observations. First, if these illnesses cannot be found in the brain, surely they cannot be 'brain diseases' – they must be something else. The second observation is really more of a question – when can we give ourselves permission to stop looking?

How does all of this relate to ADHD?

These issues are important in understanding the debate around ADHD. Pro-ADHD researchers have been extremely keen to apply these techniques to their search for the elusive neurophysiological 'proof' of this supposed disorder. This has resulted in a number of reports suggesting that neuro-imaging has, indeed, been able to demonstrate evidence that the brains of children diagnosed with ADHD are different from those of 'ordinary' children. However, this is not so, as the following examples show.

Example 1: the 'medication effect'

A review of 33 studies by US researchers, Jonathan Leo and David Cohen, in 2003 found that there was widespread failure to consider the effects of medication on the children who participated.[9] In these studies, 93% of children in the 'ADHD diagnosed' group were either taking stimulant medication, had just stopped it, or had been on it for years. Leo commented that 'Dr Cohen and I pulled the studies that had been done on brain imaging and ADHD and what jumped out at us was that every single study used medicated kids, subjects who had been on stimulants or some other drugs that we don't know because that information wasn't made part of the study.' Obviously, the fact that so many of the children had been taking drugs makes it impossible to draw any conclusions about what the findings mean. For example, do they show the effect of stimulant drug use, or 'ADHD', or something else entirely?

Example 2: the 'size effect'

In 2001, a large National Institute for Mental Health in England (NIMHE) study led by F Xavier Castellanos and known subsequently as 'the Castellanos study' conducted MRI scans on 544 children, comparing the brains of 'ADHD' children with those of a 'control group' of children who did not have the diagnosis.[10] The results were widely reported to the effect that children with ADHD had 'significantly smaller brain volumes' which were found to be unrelated to drug treatment. However, as Leo and Cohen pointed out, the two groups (ADHD and non-ADHD) were not matched for age – the non-ADHD control group was more than 2 years older than the ADHD group. As brain size is typically related to head size, and the control group was significantly taller and heavier than the ADHD group, Leo and Cohen concluded that it was hardly surprising that there were differences in brain size! In response, Castellanos commented, rather oddly, that the disparity in age reflected the fact that 'it is very difficult to find kids who are unmedicated.'[11]

In her article for *Insight* on the Leo and Cohen paper, Kelly O'Meara reported Leo as commenting that 'given all the problems with ADHD imaging research, parents who are contemplating medicating their children should not be told there is a biological basis for ADHD.'[12] In a later article, Cohen claimed that the medication issue continued to be 'wilfully obscured' by researchers.[13]

Haven't we been here before? Phrenology revisited

Critics of the claims made on behalf of anatomical and functional neuro-imaging caution against creating a 'modern-day phrenology.'[14] It might be worth reminding ourselves about phrenology, which was extremely influential in its day (*see* Box 8.3).

In some ways, neuro-imaging *is* doing the same thing that phrenology did in the past, in that it is engaged in developing maps of the brain and cerebral cortex. This is undeniably adding to our knowledge about the brain, but it also has its limitations. Maps can tell us a great deal about the physical properties of countries, such as where they are, and their shape and structure. But of course they tell us nothing about what the different countries are *like*, the people who populate them, their culture, how they live, and their relationships with themselves and with other peoples. This information is missing. Neuro-imaging is important but, as the neuroscientists know, it is not the whole story.

BOX 8.3 Phrenology

Phrenology was developed in the nineteenth century by the Viennese physician, Franz Joseph Gall. It was based on the idea that different aspects of the mind had separate and distinct 'organs' in the brain, the size of which corresponded to their power. These various organs determined the shape of the brain, which in turn influenced the contours of the skull. Phrenologists believed that the surface of the skull revealed a person's character and intellectual aptitudes. Phrenologists engaged in assessment and diagnosis, and could even be called upon to provide job references. The 'science' spread across Europe and attracted physicians and lay-persons alike. Phrenologising – head reading – became very popular during the second half of the nineteenth century, and would attract huge audiences.

We now know that there was absolutely no scientific basis to phrenology. The 'organs' identified by the phrenologists do not exist. However, their basic ideas about localisation of function have proved to have some accuracy, and recent research has confirmed that those areas of the brain that are most frequently used do indeed increase in size.[15] Proof, perhaps, that you can't make a scientific theory out of a couple of ideas. Proof also that 'testing' your theories by simply looking for more and more evidence to confirm what you believe anyway is no way to go about developing scientific credibility.

There is no substance to the claims that neuro-imaging has confirmed that ADHD is a brain disorder. Nor has any neurophysiological 'pattern' of defects or any consistent abnormality emerged. If it had, and we understood what we were looking at, we would be none the wiser – such discoveries would still leave us unable to answer 'cause-and-effect' questions.[16]

Most importantly, since we know that how children are cared for has an impact on the developing brain, there is a danger of misinterpreting what we are seeing when we look at 'snapshot' images of the brain. As we have seen, early nurturing and trauma both influence how the brain develops, as do factors like nutrition. A disproportionate number of children in poverty are exposed to factors that are known to have a detrimental influence on brain development. The evidence suggests that it is the children in these groups who are also most likely to, erroneously, be given a diagnosis of ADHD (this is discussed in more detail in Chapter 10). So when we are shown pictures highlighting the differences between 'ADHD brains' and others, what are they really showing? They could indeed be showing us something of the impact of poverty and deprivation during the early years, as well as poor attachment, neglect and abuse. The evidence could just as easily suggest these kinds of conclusions. But then they would be equally nebulous. The fact is that we just cannot tell from these studies what we are really looking at.

Where does this leave us?

The brain does not develop according to a genetically programmed blueprint. Instead, there is a complex process of adaptation, in which there appear to be periods of rapid growth, following by 'pruning' as the brain adapts to its environment. It is now believed that new synapses, or at least reorganisation of existing ones, has to be possible in order for adult learning (such as the learning of new languages) to take place. It is likely that continued adaptation to new environments requires the adding and subtracting of synapses. The neurobiologist William Calvin refers to the brain as a 'Darwin machine' that works on the principle of 'make lots of random variants by brute bashing about, and then select the good ones.'[17]

The processes by which behaviour affects the brain, and vice versa, are notoriously difficult to tease out. Theorists suggest that it is highly likely that the brain and the mind influence each other – cognitive (mental) processes are elicited by brain activity, but they also in turn cause brain activity, thus influencing the course of behaviour. The mind and the brain can therefore be described as a 'two-way street.'[18]

Curiously, clinical research has been demonstrating this for a good many years. After all, we know that psychological intervention can affect brain physiology and brain chemistry,[19] as can a placebo.[20] The literature suggests that we may be looking in the wrong place and in the wrong way if we are expecting to find neurophysiological evidence that can differentiate 'ADHD' from 'non-ADHD' brains. For those of us who do not believe that there is such a clinical construct as 'ADHD', this makes perfect sense. As Sami Timimi points out, the elements of ADHD are, at best, a disparate group of characteristics that apply to all children at one time or another.[21] What *has* emerged from these kinds of studies is not only inconsistent but also inconclusive. Rather than confirming the 'existence' of 'ADHD' in the brain, they end up doing the very opposite.

The real problem with many of the brain-imaging reports is that they have been 'talked up' and have unfortunately been easy to hijack and use as part of the oversimplified disease model touted by the biological propagandists. What I hope I have shown in this chapter is how complex brain–mind processes are, however we try to conceptualise them. What I also hope it shows is something of how problems can be in the mind but not in the brain.

As for the mind–brain relationship, the debate continues. Evidence of neuroplasticity has been seen to present a challenge to so-called 'reductionist' assumptions that psychology can be reduced to mere neurophysiological processes. If this were the case, psychological therapies would be redundant. The fact that they are not and that there is considerable evidence for their effectiveness over medication would seem to support the idea that changes in mind (and behaviour) can come first (i.e. before brain changes). At most, it seems that neuropsychological information provides functional descriptions of some psychological processes.

As a suitable end point, it is worth mentioning that the official website of the American Psychiatric Association has featured a position paper (drafted in January 2005) on the use of functional imaging technologies in children and teenagers. This paper states the following:

> Imaging research cannot yet be used to diagnose psychiatric illness, and may not be useful in clinical practice for a number of years . . . Specifically, no published investigation in the field has determined that any structural or functional abnormality is

specific to a single psychiatric disorder. Additionally, imaging studies examine groups of patients and healthy controls; therefore, findings may not apply to all individuals with a given disorder. Even when significant differences are identified between groups, there is a substantial overlap among individuals in both groups . . . We conclude that, at the present time, the available evidence does not support the use of brain imaging for clinical diagnosis or treatment of psychiatric disorders.[22]

There is an issue where 'looking for proof' is concerned, since it is the very thing that scientists mustn't do. There are an unlimited number of events out there that can provide supportive evidence for a theory. That is why scientific studies do not attempt to prove a theory – they look to disprove it. For this, we need only a single piece of evidence. To do anything else really does make us no better than the phrenologists.

Grace Jackson, who is not only a psychiatrist but also an expert on neuro-imaging, deserves the final word. She writes:

Contrary to the reports which have been emphasised by the major news outlets, there is no evidence at this time to justify the claim that brain scans discern the presence of psychiatric disease, based upon anatomic or physiological abnormalities of the brain. For a variety of theoretical and practical limitations, the functioning imaging technologies . . . cannot reliably predict the presence of psychopathology. For philosophical reasons, it is highly doubtful that they ever will.[23]

CHAPTER 9

Choice for children?

The story so far . . .

As we have seen, ADHD remains a controversial diagnosis. Does it exist at all? Or are we just re-labelling other difficulties that children might have (not to mention ordinary naughtiness) as ADHD? There are two distinct 'camps' – 'believers' and 'non-believers' – whose views tend to be broadly split according to their beliefs about human behaviour and mental health. These beliefs tend to be polarised around whether biological or psychosocial influences should be emphasised in children's lives (a variant of the perennial 'nature–nurture' debate). The fact that the evidence for a biological disorder remains equivocal does nothing to resolve this argument. The water is further muddied by the drug companies, who have their own agendas. (Their involvement has been described in earlier chapters.)

The perceptive reader might protest at this point at my positioning of people on either one side or the other of this ideological 'fence.' And of course they have a point. There are those who claim the middle ground – 'it's a bit of both' – but on close examination we have to ask ourselves whether this is a tenable position. The philosophical differences between these two models of mental health, in my opinion, make a nonsense of the idea that you can simply graft one on to another.

The 'bit-of-both' explanation has, for years, enabled the dominant biological view to continue to regard the rest of human experience as a mere add-on. It softens the hard biological dogma and makes it acceptable, rather than revealing it as something to be challenged. You see, where we stand in this debate really does matter. It influences, among other things, the position that we take about what kind of help is needed. In short, either we are talking about something that is a biological condition or we are not. So far, despite years of research and incredible amounts of money being spent trying to prove the opposite, it seems that we are *not*. But this is neither the message that is heard by the general public nor that heard by those who have the power to determine how mental health and social care resources are allocated.

How we understand problems

Previous chapters have presented something of the wider debate around ADHD and, in particular, some of the *environmental* influences on children that might lead them to behave in ways that attract medical labels of one disorder or another. In a way, these children's problems can be likened to an iceberg floating in the sea. Only a fraction of it is visible, while the rest – the majority of the iceberg – is beneath the water and effectively hidden from view. Unfortunately, whatever claims individuals might make, biological approaches focus on symptoms – the tip of the iceberg – *at the expense of other considerations*. A child who comes to the clinic feeling 'depressed' will have the depression treated and, if they are treated by a medic (or a medical team), will most probably receive medication if the depression is deemed to be in the clinical range. But what has led to the depression?

Gaining an understanding of this will help us to address the *real* problem, which is not that the child is 'depressed', but *what is causing them to feel depressed*. This is the complex part of the iceberg that lies beneath the water and shows itself in the symptoms. This is why most sensible therapists, regardless of their particular therapeutic approach, would seek to work with the child's family, rather than just with the child. And this is why most sensible therapists would be asking themselves, on meeting a supposedly 'ADHD child', 'What is underneath this "attention problem"? What else is going on and what does all this mean?' Only after understanding this can we begin to help to address some of the real problems. Ultimately, we need to remember that symptoms are not everything. They are only a small part of the picture – literally, the tip of the iceberg.

We need to make absolutely sure that we understand what has contributed to children's difficulties, and that we take time to explore and understand the meaning of their behaviour. If we focus only on symptoms, we risk not only becoming ineffective helpers, but also making things worse.

'Blaming the child'

Biological/medical approaches often stop at the description – or diagnosis – of the problem. This in turn determines the 'treatment' that is needed. Although mental health teams offer a range of therapies and treatments, *if your starting point is the premise that a child has a biological illness, they are not going to make much difference*. This is because, whatever you do, you will be acting on the assumption that it is the child who has the 'disorder.' Everything you do after making such a diagnosis has this as its frame of reference. This fact alone changes everything that comes afterwards.

This leads to a situation where children can, in effect, be blamed for the difficulties in their lives. The child who experiences chronic family problems, family breakdown, abuse or neglect translates as 'the ADHD child.' The child who lives in deprived circumstances and who suffers harsh and inconsistent parenting is 'conduct disordered.' We so often fail to address children's problems because we are too busy labelling them as disordered. When we do this, it absolves us of our responsibilities as adults – especially parents, who are so effectively absolved of their responsibilities *if the problem is really the child and not them.* Let's revisit the story of Kurt Cobain (*see* Box 9.1).

BOX 9.1 Back to Kurt Cobain*

Kurt Cobain was a troubled boy from a troubled family. His childhood was characterised by family breakdown, emotional and physical abuse, neglect, rejection, family drug and alcohol use, and domestic violence. A number of family members committed suicide. He was a boy who drifted between family and friends, and who at one time slept in a cardboard box on his friend's porch. The degree of disturbance in his family background can only be glimpsed between the lines of Charles Cross's biography – but like most of our lives it is what lies between the lines that tells the real story. Cross records that in June 1976, Kurt wrote on his bedroom wall 'I hate Mom, I hate Dad. Dad hates Mom, Mom hates Dad. It simply makes you want to be so sad.' At the age of 10, he was so stressed that he developed an involuntary twitching in his eyes and was admitted to hospital with what family members described as 'malnutrition.' At the age of 11, Cross tells the reader, Kurt's behaviour led to school and then family concerns. In addition to becoming more defiant of adult authority, he had started bullying another boy at school. And the solution to this? Kurt's parents didn't look at their own behaviour and its impact and influence on him. Instead they concluded that he needed counselling.

No matter that he was living with violence and bullying himself – the decision was made that there was something wrong with Kurt, and he was the one who needed 'fixing.' Like many retrospective accounts in which the central character commits suicide, there is a theme running through the book to the effect that there was always something 'wrong' with Kurt. This really does depend on which lens you happen to be looking through. Some readers might remember the Munsters, the TV family of freaks who had their non-freaky niece living with them. One of the comedy themes running through the show was how they pitied this beautiful girl for her 'ugliness.'

Kurt Cobain's history is not unique. On the contrary, it is depressingly common. If you work with children it can make you want to shout out loud 'Well, what did you think would happen?' Of course, we're never allowed to say this.

Not all parents want to blame their children for what happens to them and, thankfully, there are plenty of parents who are ready to work at making changes, wherever these changes need to be made. What of them? What do children's services offer them? The fact is that it can be extremely difficult for parents and carers to access help, whether at home or at school (for children and young people themselves, of course, it is almost impossible).

■ It is increasingly difficult to access social work support – even for families who are under considerable stress.

■ It is increasingly difficult to obtain respite care for children with disabilities so that their parents can take a break.

---

* From information provided in Cross CR. *Heavier than Heaven: the biography of Kurt Cobain.* London: Hodder and Stoughton; 2001.

- It is increasingly difficult to secure educational support.
- It is not difficult to obtain Ritalin.

Perhaps this is one of the reasons why Ritalin prescribing has mushroomed as it has. Whereas other forms of help have become increasingly difficult to access, medication is easy to obtain. It offers, on the face of it, a 'quick-fix' solution. It offers other benefits, too.

- Schools can access additional resources if they have children with mental health diagnoses, such as ADHD.
- Parents are eligible for Disability Living Allowance if their child has an ADHD diagnosis. (If you're on a low income, this helps. It is also hard to give up, once you have it.)
- Parents have a 'peg' on which to hang their child's difficult behaviour. This peg is labelled 'See? It wasn't us.'
- The child has an excuse for any bad behaviour. This goes something like 'See? It's not me, it's my ADHD.'
- Mental health services, already under enormous pressures and often lacking practitioners with the skills necessary to address these children's difficulties, can create a 'fast-track' treatment programme which involves little more than regular monitoring and prescribing.

Everyone's a winner. Or so it might have seemed.

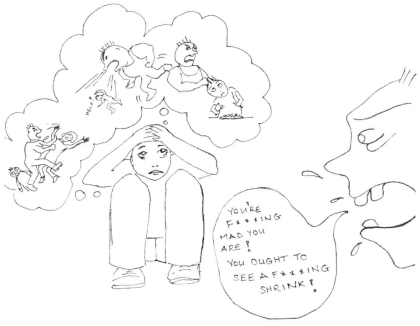

FIGURE 9.1 'You're mad, you are.'

So what's happened . . .?

In the event, what seemed initially to be the solution (to the ADHD issue) has now become the problem. Hard-pressed GPs and mental health teams have found themselves with rising numbers of children diagnosed with ADHD *who won't go away*. They have discovered that many of these children do not just take their Ritalin and go quietly – their families actually expect them to get better. So they keep coming back. Owing to the fact that their problems have been mislabelled and remain untreated, they often ricochet around the system, to no avail. Health workers start to resent these 'problem families.' Psychiatrists resent their 'Ritalin clinics', often inherited from other, ADHD-enthusiast consultants, where they are simply required to process these children. As for the cost of all this medication, it has also mushroomed. The bill for hyperactivity drugs in England is in excess of £10 million a year. I'm not sure exactly what kinds of other services this amount of money could buy for children, but I do know that this is *10 times* the budget for Specialist Children's Services in the Trust where I work, and *double* the budget for the entire Children's Directorate. By my estimate, it would buy about 270,000 extra psychologists, family therapists or specialist nurses, who could work with children and families using proven psychological methods that do not require drugs.

Alternatives to Ritalin

In my clinic in South Staffordshire, where I worked until 2005, we had an interesting situation. Like many healthcare providers, our services are divided into 'patches', or localities, that correspond to geographical areas. We found that while some areas were recording incidences of over 100 children with ADHD, the figure in my clinic 20 miles down the road was zero. Now if we accept that these children are not going to differ drastically from one part of this fairly small geographical area to another, we must also ask ourselves why there was such variation in the incidence of ADHD. Having journeyed this far into the book, you will already know the answer. The answer lies in how these children's difficulties were understood and responded to.

In my own clinic, we understood the differences in numbers of diagnoses to reflect three major factors. The first was the particular culture of the mental health teams (i.e. how they view children's problems). The second factor was what type of professionals were in the teams (whether they were trained according to a so-called medical/biological model or a psychosocial one). The third factor was what type of skills the professionals in each team had at their disposal.

A tale of two clinics

Perhaps not surprisingly, my experience of children's mental health teams across the region in which I worked has been that those made up largely or exclusively of medical personnel, such as doctors and nurses, tended to have more children diagnosed with ADHD. In contrast, teams containing psychologists, family counsellors and psychologically trained social workers would make very few of these diagnoses – if any.

You might well suggest that it could be a lack of medical training that prevents this kind of team from making ADHD diagnoses (in other words, they are not correctly diagnosing these children), but you would be mistaken. My own clinical team had a visiting psychiatrist who concurred with our views. Although we had trained medical personnel we did not have a *medical culture*, which is important. What was different was that we adopted a good practice model that did not channel the child directly down a medical route as soon as the phrase 'ADHD' was mentioned in a referral letter. Instead, it was business as usual – together with the child, their family and school, we took a close look at what was going on and how we could help. It wasn't a case of 'assessing for ADHD', or even of 'ruling out ADHD' – we simply didn't arrive at that point. Having looked very closely at all aspects of the difficulties presented to us, we found that our 'care pathway' took us nowhere near the road labelled 'ADHD.' It took us elsewhere.

The other clinic, in contrast, had opened an 'ADHD Clinic' to fast-track children who were thought to have this condition. There was soon a huge number of young people with a diagnosis of ADHD coming to the clinic, where they were put on medication and monitored at regular intervals. This approach resulted in a substantial drugs bill, as well as a monthly 'heartsink' clinic that none of the professionals really wanted to do. It would be unfair to suggest that this was all that happened. I understand additional work was sometimes offered to the family ('parenting work', in particular), but this was as an adjunct to the drug treatment, which had been set up as the main intervention for these youngsters. What was important was that the 'frame of reference' for the parents, teachers and child was that *it was the child who had the 'disorder.'* Were the two systems compared? They were never compared formally, which is a pity, although some comparisons were drawn 'informally.' And what was the result? I was accused of depriving children of their Ritalin.

We would all agree that it is unacceptable that what is offered in one area can differ so much from that which is available in another, yet this kind of picture has been replicated across the country for years – not just in relation to ADHD, but in terms of healthcare in general. This is one of the areas flagged up by government that must change. The current emphasis is not only on equitability and quality standards, but also on choice. However, the government focus on standardising care through the use of algorithms such as the NICE guidelines threatens to lead to a more, rather than less, medicalised approach. I don't know if any of our families were disenchanted with what they were offered and simply went elsewhere to get their Ritalin. They might well have done. But if they did, we were unaware of it. The important thing is that at least they had a choice. If you find yourself on the medical conveyor belt you will probably never even realise that there *is* a choice.

The reality of the situation is that there is only a limited amount of money available for healthcare. Therefore what is spent on drugs cannot be spent on other resources. For many mental health workers this means that there are not enough workers to do the job. Never mind the skills – there are just not enough pairs of hands. Properly resourced, many children's services could easily offer alternatives to drug treatment that would also be cost-effective. The problem is that this would require a shift in thinking, from 'quick fix' to longer term. It also requires a commitment to *invest to save*. This means getting things right at the earliest opportunity (even though it carries a cost), so that savings can be made later on – in every sense of the word. These are radical ideas for health, social care and education, where a long-term view is rare and is made increasingly difficult by constant changes of policy and focus.

Choice and consent

In 2000, psychologist Steve Baldwin published the results of a survey in which he had asked parents and carers a series of questions about their children's treatment once they had received a diagnosis of ADHD.[1] He also asked them about the drugs that their children had been prescribed. These questions included the following:

■ Were you told about the side-effects of MPH (Ritalin) and the fact that it is an amphetamine?

■ Were you offered any non-drug alternative to MPH?

   He reported that 100% of respondents replied 'no' to both questions.

Between 2002 and 2003, a colleague of mine, Scott Sinclair, and his assistant, George Harris, replicated Steve Baldwin's survey of parents and carers who were in contact with ADHD clinics in three different locations in South Staffordshire.[2]

BOX 9.2 South Staffordshire Healthcare NHS Trust Parent/Carer Survey (2003)

What recommendations were made after your child was assessed?

■ 59%   medication only
■ 13%   medication and behaviour management
■ 7%   medication and educational support
■ 19%   non-medical intervention.

(In total, 79% of children were prescribed medication.)

These results were consistent with Steve Baldwin's 2000 survey, which found that 80% of children with a diagnosis of ADHD were put on medication. In Baldwin's study all parents reported side-effects in their children.

   Sinclair and Harris (2003) then asked parents another question.

BOX 9.3 South Staffordshire Healthcare NHS Trust Parent/Carer Survey (2003)

What problem do you think your child has?

■ 11.3%   ADHD
■ 67%   ADHD and symptoms of other problem(s)
■ 21%   other problems.

In other words, 78% of parents and carers thought that a diagnosis of ADHD did not fully take account of their child's problems.

These responses suggest that the vast majority of children who attend mental health clinics will be prescribed stimulant medication, most probably Ritalin. For most of them, research shows that this will be their *only* intervention. This is despite the fact that most of their parents believe that 'ADHD' is only a partial explanation for their children's problems. This latter finding strongly suggests, among other things, that some mental health professionals may be seizing on 'attention' as a primary problem (and treating it) when, as discussed earlier, it is not 'the problem' at all, but merely a symptom of any one of a number of things that might be going on for the child.

Why should we be concerned?

Surveys like these confirm a predominantly medical response to children's symptoms of attentional problems, with little or no 'alternative' kind of help offered. In many cases, survey responses showed that there were no concurrent psychological programmes at all.

This is important because, as we have already seen, children may be maintained for a considerable number of years on medication that we are unsure about in terms of its effect on the biochemistry of young developing brains. Most importantly, however, there is evidence to suggest that although medication may subdue the child, it has no effect on other aspects of functioning, such as academic or psychosocial functioning.[3] This is hardly surprising. As all good psychological therapists know, *the pill does not teach the skill.*

Teaching 'the skill'

And yet we *can* help to develop these skills in children and young people. Some of us have been doing it for years, using tried and tested psychological methods. Rather than using medication as a 'first-line' treatment, shouldn't we be doing more of this? Assuming that there really are children who have these difficulties without any complex underlying problems, surely it would be far better to help them to develop much-needed self-regulation skills. Many of us already support children in this way, both in the school environment and at home if necessary. This means that they can have successful experiences at school, rather than aversive ones and, furthermore, that they have these skills for life. If this approach was available for parents – and children – what would they choose? After all, as the psychologist David Keirsey puts it, 'Just because physicians are not trained to treat behaviour is no reason for them to assume others aren't.'[4]

We should be concerned that parents are being offered little or no choice – certainly not *informed* choice. But there is something we should be even more concerned about. What choices are we offering our children?

Choice for children

The issue of choice for children is an important one. For a number of years, mental health services have struggled with the issue of who is their client. Services in the UK used to be called 'Child Guidance Clinics', which at least made it clear that it was the parent who was the client. Nowadays it's all a bit of a mix-up. Although most services claim to place the child at their centre, it is invariably the concerns of the parent that gain priority over those of the child (if you are in any doubt about this, ask yourself who is sent the satisfaction questionnaire). With regard to formal consent to treatment, this is rarely obtained. Some consultants have expressed the view to me that 'turning up to appointments' is evidence of consent. On one occasion, when I raised the issue of *informed* consent in relation to Ritalin, I was given the answer that the leaflet produced by the drug company accompanying the medication constituted sufficient 'information' for parents. It is a fact that very little information is given to children and families about the side-effects or long-term risks of taking stimulant medication. Furthermore, *it is not unknown for children to be taking Ritalin without their knowledge* (*see* Box 9.4).

BOX 9.4 The case of the sneaky medication

An assistant psychologist told me about one of the training cases she was given, involving an 11-year-old boy who had a diagnosis of ADHD. He had been referred back to the service after his mother told their GP that the family was on the point of breaking up because of his bad behaviour. During the course of her first meeting with the family, the assistant psychologist mentioned the boy's medication and discovered that this had been a secret from him for 4 years. His parents had given it to him surreptitiously, without him ever knowing he was taking it. When she reported this to her supervisor, he was angry with her for her lack of preparation for the appointment – if she had read the file as thoroughly as she should have, she would have known that the boy was unaware that he was being medicated, as it was clearly recorded.*

This boy had certainly never given his consent to drug treatment. My guess is that his parents must have known that he would not be happy with it, otherwise why would they have resorted to such trickery?

When this story was relayed to me, I was alarmed to hear that this kind of practice could occur and that clinic staff seemed to be colluding with it. I began to wonder how many more children out there were taking these drugs against their wishes. This again raised for me the issue of informed consent. For those whose consent has been sought, do they really know what they are taking? Do they know that there are non-drug alternatives (230 alternative psychological and social therapies, none of which involve medication, according to Steve Baldwin).[5]

The more I thought about this, the more it seemed to me to make a mockery of the idea of consent and 'choice' (so beloved of the NHS reformers). This most vulnerable

---

* Assistant psychologist, personal communication, 2003.

group of society is at the mercy of several 'tiers' of adults, who make decisions on their behalf. Although, ironically, the child is effectively the 'client' (or patient) who is registered with the mental health clinic, he or she is rarely included in the decision making. It is a question of being 'told' what to do, not asked what they would like to do.

Similarly, scant attention is paid to how diagnoses like 'ADHD' make children feel.

> **BOX 9.5 On being considered 'normal' . . .**
>
> I met a young man who had recently moved to the area. He had already been given a diagnosis of ADHD and had been medicated, with little or no effect. His mother had brought him to the clinic because she was finding him unmanageable. This mother and son had had an extremely difficult few years. As I often do, at the end of our meeting I reflected aloud on what we had talked about. I commented on what the family had been through and, directly to the young man, what he had personally been through, adding that he 'would just not be normal' if he hadn't responded with the degree of distress that he had. He became tearful and responded that this was the first time in years someone had said he was normal.

Peter Breggin is exceptional in focusing on how Ritalin makes children feel. He comments that 'The youngsters I have talked to have felt that Ritalin put them "out of touch" and made them "feel weird", blunting their feelings and subduing them.' Breggin goes on to cite an unpublished study by three doctors, Peter Jensen, Michael Bain and Allen Josephson, who researched what children thought about taking medication. They found that many children thought they were taking their tablets to 'control' them because they were 'bad.' The researchers also found that children who were taking medication tended to blame their behaviour on 'outside sources', such as eating sugar or not taking their pill. They did not attribute any responsibility to themselves.[6]

Pressure and intimidation

It is now common for mental health professionals to receive referrals from schools, or at least initiated by schools, where a child has been excluded and will not be readmitted 'until he has a diagnosis' and is receiving 'treatment' (presumably by this they mean stimulant medication). I have met a number of parents who have been bullied in this way into going along with what they felt was against their better judgement.

One of these was Cathy, who was pressured into seeking a diagnosis for her son, Alex (who, incidentally, already had a diagnosis of Asperger's syndrome). Cathy started Alex on medication, but was so upset by the effect it had on him that she discontinued it. She told me that Alex's teacher had called her a 'bad mother' for taking her son off medication, and had told her they had no alternative but to exclude him. Obliged to obtain a mental health referral for her son because she wanted to keep him in school, Cathy found herself seeing me. She had been so worried about what might happen and what might be said to her that she didn't come to her first appointment. She arrived late for her second one, telling me 'I nearly didn't come at all.'

Cathy explained to me that she had no problems at all managing Alex's behaviour at home. Her description of him was that of a happy, much-loved adolescent, albeit 'quirky.' He had a passion for cars, and was building a kit-car with his father. His parents seemed to manage his behaviour well. What came across to me most strongly was that they really seemed to value their son's uniqueness. Alex was known to be a bit of a character, but was well liked in the village where the family lived. Exploration suggested that his behaviour had never been much of problem at school until there had been a change in his weekday routine (Alex had a part-time timetable in two different schools). Following this, he had become 'uncooperative' with his teachers and disruptive during some of his lessons. His mother understood this to be explained by his Asperger's syndrome, reasoning that children with this constellation of difficulties do best when their environments are routine and predictable. What seemed to have driven the situation in Alex's case was a kind of power struggle between the parents and the school. As Alex was in his final year at school and Cathy knew that she hadn't got years of disagreements to face, it was not difficult for her to be assertive about her son's needs, especially since she had 'complied' with the school's insistence that she should come to see me.

Other parents and other children, I am sure, have not been so fortunate.

Lack of availability of 'talking therapies'

In recent years, considerable media attention has been given to depression and antidepressants. In particular, the focus has been on the ease with which antidepressant medication has been prescribed, and the corresponding difficulty of accessing non-medical treatment, such as psychological therapies. This has been despite the fact that some psychological therapies (e.g. cognitive behavioural therapy) have a proven track record of effectiveness. By way of explanation, a number of newspaper articles have cited the unfavourable 'cost' of psychological therapies as the determining factor, which should come as a surprise to those of us who work within the mental health system, and who see this as an issue of neither cost nor availability, but of dominant culture, priorities and power.

At the same time as thousands of prescriptions for drugs are being written because there are too few therapists, we are told in the recent report by Lord Layard that there are many people who receive no help at all because they feel that drugs are not for them.[7] For them, there is no alternative. They are denied access to psychological therapies because there are insufficient numbers of trained psychologists and psychological therapists.

For children, who seem never to be worth mentioning in any of these reports, the situation is worse. As we have already seen, they are unlikely to be the decision makers in their own treatment, and equally unlikely to understand what is happening and why. For years there has been an appalling lack of choice and lack of availability of alternatives to medical treatment for children who have been given a diagnosis of 'ADHD.' We already know that these children are likely to have a complex set of problems, and that (like others) they can be helped by a *multi-systemic* approach (psychological therapies that span educational, family and community domains), but few children are able to access such a holistic approach. We need to ask ourselves whether a diagnosis of 'ADHD' is helpful to these children in these circumstances, or whether a comprehensive understanding and description of their difficulties – more like a psychological formulation – is more likely to secure them the help that they need. However, here's the catch. If we allow that such a description might serve so-called 'ADHD children' better than a medical diagnosis, we might have to think of it being better for other children, too.

And here's another catch, or rather a question. What do we think of a supposedly biological problem that can be *entirely alleviated* by a psychosocial approach? Using the kind of medical reasoning that we discussed in Chapter 1, we might ask why such evidence isn't seen as 'proof' of its psychosocial origin. If we could be so bold – if we could speak with the same kind of authority as the advocates of biological psychiatry – we would years ago have called for a psychosocial system of describing people's problems to replace the biological one. Why haven't we done this? Peter Breggin suggests one important reason:

> Psychiatry and psychiatrists must not be allowed to make false claims about the genetic and biological origins of so-called mental illness. Such claims are unethical, if not fraudulent, and serve only to perpetuate the influence of the profession and individual practitioners. But if it rejected its biopsychiatric claims, the profession would admit to being something very difficult to justify or defend – a medical specialty that does not treat medical illnesses.[8]

CHAPTER 10

Social and political issues

The social context of mental health

Worldwide, it is a fact that poor people are more likely than rich people to become ill and die earlier. It is common for those of us living in wealthier countries to be told that there is not much 'absolute' poverty any more – what now exists is 'relative' poverty. In other words, the poor are not really poor – standards have risen to mean that their lives are impoverished only in relation to those of other citizens, whose standards of living have improved by a greater margin. It might come as a surprise therefore to hear that research shows the health of the poor is affected not by absolute poverty but by *the size of the gap between rich and poor*. According to the *British Medical Journal*, 'what matters in determining mortality and health in society is less the overall wealth of that society and more how evenly wealth is distributed.'[1] The distribution of wealth seems to determine other benefits, too, such as spending on education and income support, which means that the greater the inequality of income, the more likely people are to be unemployed, imprisoned and poorly educated. The 'wealth gap' looks to be a fairly robust formula that can be applied across countries.[*]

Mental health problems are also more common in adults who live in disadvantaged circumstances. Studies show that people who are poor are much more likely to be suffering from poor mental health. This risk is even greater if they are socially excluded.[2] Although specific mental health problems seem to arise from a complex interaction of factors, their distribution maps neatly on to social factors, such as culture, social class, age, ethnicity and gender.[3]

Many who work in mental health services are struck by the lack of emphasis given to the social conditions of their service users. One such person is Mark Bertram, an occupational therapist and vocational service manager in Lambeth, London. Mark says, 'Most of the work my colleagues engage in is focused on trying to help people

---

[*] On the same website, Peter Montague, in his essay, 'Economic inequality and health', cites the following studies: Kaplan GA *et al.* Inequality in income and mortality in the United States: analysis of mortality and potential pathways. *BMJ.* 1996; **312**: 999–1003. Kennedy B *et al.* Income distribution and mortality: cross-sectional ecological study of the Robin Hood Index in the United States. *BMJ.* 1996; **312**: 1004–7. Wilkinson RG. Income distribution and life expectancy. *BMJ.* 1992; **304**: 165–8. Waldmann RJ. Income distribution and infant mortality. *Q J Economics.* 1992; **107**: 1283–302.

clobbered and disabled by the miserable effects of poverty and deprivation within a shaming benefits system and discriminating society.' His experiences of mental health work are described in Box 10.1.

> ### BOX 10.1 Reflections of a mental health worker
>
> I work in mental health services in an area that has the highest level of violent street crime nationally, very high levels of socio-economic deprivation, unemployment, drug abuse and 'psychiatric morbidity.' It has been described in the press and through graffiti as a war zone, ghetto and dumping ground.
>
> To use the same analogies, the people I meet appear to be living examples of social inequality and the seriously wounded casualties. In my experience over 14 years, the people I work with tell stories about their experience of distress that are entirely understandable in the lived oppressive context of what has happened to them. The key point is that many 'have been done to or neglected' and have suffered the impact of gross inequalities to the extent that they cannot cope any more. Many consistently describe struggling with extreme emotional and social deprivation, abuse, traumas and a lack of educational or vocational opportunity.[4]

When people write about marginalised groups, they usually neglect to mention children, who are most vulnerable of all. What about children's mental health? What are the lessons from research about their living circumstances?

The social context of children's mental health

One recent document that has looked at the prevalence of 'mental disorders' and social circumstances is the Department of Health's *Mental Health of Children and Young People in Great Britain, 2004*.[5] This report outlines a number of factors that are implicated in children's mental health difficulties. They are worth repeating here.

The survey found that 'mental disorders' were more common in children:

- living with a lone parent
- living in reconstituted families
- whose interviewed parent had no educational qualifications
- living in families where neither parent was working
- living in families with a gross weekly household income of less than £100
- living in households in which someone received disability benefit
- living in families where the household reference person was in a routine occupational group compared with those with a reference person in the higher professional group
- living in the social or privately rented sector compared with those who owned accommodation
- living in areas classed as 'hard pressed' compared with areas classed as 'wealthy achievers' or 'urban prosperity.'

These findings again raise the question of exactly what we are measuring when we set out to measure 'mental disorder.' Many of the above categories are indications of social deprivation and disadvantage, while some are also indicators of family instability, which is known to be a continuing stressful condition for children. When we talk about 'mental disorder' and try to measure it, it seems that time and time again we end up with a constellation of behaviours that are – to continue to use this medical language – *symptoms* of deprivation, poor parenting, trauma, family breakdown, repeated experiences of separation and loss, and the chronic stress that arises from all of these factors. So are we really measuring mental health disorders or are we measuring the effects of disadvantage?

One thing seems certain. These statistics confirm that social deprivation and stressful conditions are not good for children. In addition to the many problems they create, they also lead to emotional problems that are severe enough to warrant special help – those classed here as 'mental health disorders.' The logical solution to this reasoning, you might think, would be to try to take steps to alleviate the conditions that compromise children's psychological well-being. But we don't do this. Instead, we choose to call their difficulties 'disorders', and we focus on 'treating' them. The implication is that children who live in disadvantaged circumstances have behaviours and psychological difficulties that are *abnormal*. Is this really the case? Experience tells us just the opposite. Many of us who work with children on a daily basis see, on the contrary, troubled children who are *perfectly adjusted* to environments that are steeped in problems. It is their environments that are abnormal – not the children.

Children who have emotional problems

Let us continue with the report, *Mental Health of Children and Young People in Great Britain, 2004*, which goes on to summarise its findings in relation to children's 'emotional disorders.' The survey reported that children who had a parent with serious mental illness or families that were 'dysfunctional' were more likely to have 'emotional disorders' themselves, and over half (55%) of children with an emotional disorder had experienced their parents' separation.

In other words, the emotional environment in which the child lives has an all-important influence on his or her emotional well-being.

Children with 'conduct disorder'

The same survey also reports on the environmental characteristics of children classified as having 'conduct disorders.'* This group of children is reported to:

---

* Conduct disorder is defined by the American Academy of Child and Adolescent Psychiatry as 'a group of behavioural and emotional problems in youngsters. Children and adolescents with this disorder have great difficulty following rules and behaving in a socially acceptable way. They are often viewed by other children, adults and social agencies as 'bad' or delinquent, rather than mentally ill. Many factors may contribute to a child developing conduct disorder, including brain damage, child abuse, genetic vulnerability, school failure and traumatic life experiences.' Further details can be found at www.aacap.org/page.ww?mane=Conduct+Disorder/&Section=Facts+for+Families

- be living with cohabiting, single or previously married lone parents
- be living in households where there are large numbers of children
- have a large number of siblings
- be more likely to have parents with no educational qualifications
- be more likely to live in the most economically disadvantaged circumstances.

The above factors would suggest to many that the environments of children who are labelled as 'conduct-disordered' are those least conducive to good parenting. When parents have problems managing their children's behaviour, for whatever reasons, their children are likely to have behaviour – or 'conduct' – problems.

Children with hyperkinetic disorders

The term 'hyperkinetic' is used to describe so-called disorders of overactivity and includes, in this piece of research, ADHD. For those children classed as having hyperkinetic disorder (HKD), the following factors emerged from the survey data.

- Two-thirds of children with HKD also had a concurrent diagnosis of conduct disorder.
- Children with HKD were predominantly boys.
- Children with HKD were more likely than other children to be living with single or previously married lone parents.
- Over a third (36%) of children with HKD had parents with no formal educational qualifications.
- Over half (52%) of children with HKD lived in households with a gross weekly income of less than £300.
- The proportion of children with HKD living in a household in which no parent was working was over twice that among children with no such disorder.
- Children with HKD were more likely than other children to live in households in which someone received a disability benefit.
- Over two-fifths (43%) of parents of children with HKD had a score on the General Health Questionnaire (GHQ-12) indicative of an emotional disorder.
- Over a third (36%) of families containing children with HKD were assessed as having unhealthy family functioning.
- Almost half (49%) of children with HKD had experienced their parents' separation, and almost a quarter (23%) had had a serious mental illness that required a stay in hospital.

What this kind of information demonstrates is the how the types of adversity, culture and parenting experienced by children and young people map on to the problems that emerge for them at the other end. There are no surprises here. Young people's emotional health is adversely affected when their parent(s) have emotional problems, such as anxiety and depression. They have behaviour – or conduct – problems when home conditions are poor and militate against good parenting. They have what are termed 'hyperkinetic disorders' when *both* sets of conditions occur. In other words, children who are behaviourally and emotionally compromised are most likely to live in families where there are multiple adverse conditions. This fits with what we already know about chronic stress and its effect on children and the importance of good and consistent parenting. It isn't rocket science, it isn't even science – it's common sense.

Here we come to the fundamental difference between the psychosocial and the medical (biological) model. If the difficulties experienced by children arise from their social circumstances and are the result of their adverse experiences, how can they be 'disorders' in the way that the disease model of mental health would have us believe? And, as we touched on in the previous chapter, how is it that these so-called 'disorders' can be 'cured' by attending *only* to the psychosocial aspects of their problems, rather than to the imagined biological processes that biological psychiatry *tells* us lie beneath? Perhaps we need to revisit the term 'disorder' to try to find an answer to this question.

On the use of the term 'disorder'

My computer thesaurus tells me that the term 'disorder' is synonymous with illness, sickness and disease. Another meaning equates it with chaos (as in *dis-order*). My copy of the *Oxford Compact English Dictionary* (1996 edition) confirms the 'disease' definition. Neither tool defines it in terms of problems arising from social circumstances.

The document, *Mental Health of Children and Young People in Great Britain, 2004*, like much of the mental health literature at the moment, struggles with how to position itself, and it is this struggle that is reflected in its terminology. Since the established view of mental health problems is the biological one, the language of medicine has been adopted almost universally. But this language does not quite match what has emerged from experience. Although for years there has been a sustained effort to demonstrate commonality across approaches to mental health, there is not quite the consensus that some would have us believe. What this Department of Health document does, like many others before it, is to reveal a clumsy attempt to please everyone by grafting one model of mental health on to another. This can be illustrated by the report stating (in an apparent attempt to please the non-medical contingent) that the term disorder 'should not be taken to indicate that the problem is entirely within the child.'

Confused? You might well be. They go on to say that 'Disorders arise for a variety of reasons, often interacting. In certain circumstances, a mental disorder, which describes a constellation or syndrome of features, may indicate the reactions of a young person to external circumstances, which, if changed, could largely resolve the problem.'

And here we come to the core of the argument. Exactly when was it that we came to believe it was acceptable to describe the consequences of adverse life experiences as 'mental disorders'? How can we possibly justify using such a label, when by doing so we locate the problem fairly and squarely within the child and away from any 'external circumstances', as the Department of Health report euphemistically describes them?

We make a choice when we decide to view problems in this way. We choose to accept the way things are and to believe that children's difficulties are the result of them being in some way 'faulty.' It has always been easier to fix the person rather than the environment. It also stops us asking the difficult questions, such as what our taxes are being spent on and what stops us spending public money on resolving the problems that are leading to adverse circumstances for us and our children.

Generally, however, we don't want to think about these things at all. Most of us just want to get on with our lives and have others do the thinking for us. We just want to be happy.

The imperative to be happy – and why we are so keen to 'blame the victim'

At a time when we are telling ourselves that 'mental disorders' have reached epidemic proportions, the social imperative to be happy seems never to have been greater. (The conspiracists among us might see some connections between the two.) The 'catchphrase' for modern living might best be encapsulated by the Bobby McFerrin song, 'Don't worry – be happy.'* Today's world encourages us all to focus on our own happiness and not to worry about things. Unfortunately, this can serve as a powerful injunction against thinking, as well as fostering a culture in which problems are deemed to come only to those who deserve them. In other words, life's OK – and if you have a problem there must be something wrong with you.

This is part of a well-known tendency that we all have to 'blame the victim' when bad things happen (*see* Box 10.2).

> **BOX 10.2 The Just World hypothesis**
>
> The Just World hypothesis refers to one of the ways that people make sense of the world in which they live. The theory was suggested by a social psychologist called Melvin Lerner during the 1960s. Basically it proposes that 'individuals have a need to believe they live in a world where people generally get what they deserve and deserve what they get.'[6] This way of thinking is evident in our day-to-day lives, whenever we are faced with events and circumstances that we need to process and make sense of. It predicts that we will attribute success in life to 'having deserved it' and, conversely, we will attribute misfortune to the person concerned having done something to bring it upon him- or herself. For example, the rape victim 'must have asked for it', just as the rich man 'must have deserved it.'

It could be said that mechanisms such as advertising (as well as much television programming) encourage and amplify this tendency, by promoting a view that the advantages of life are available to all, if only we can work hard enough. Alongside this runs an idea that we *should* be happy. The imperative to be happy has driven many people to seek mental health support, not because they are depressed but because they are not happy (enough). And what is the result? A great many people on Prozac who are in fact completely normal (i.e. miserable sometimes) and have no depressive illness whatsoever.

---

* Bobby McFerrin wrote the song 'Don't worry – be happy', which was a hit in the 1980s and has been used since in a number of advertisements and even in George Bush's election campaign, until McFerrin himself objected to it.

Worries that we might not be as happy as we should be run alongside other worries that we are not confident, energetic, relaxed or sexually potent enough. This is a concern that scientific journals, as well as the press, have become alerted to. For example, in an article on 'disease-mongering' published on 11 April 2006, *The Guardian* newspaper reported on concerns that 'healthy people are being turned into patients' as a result of drug company promotion of newly discovered illnesses.

The article makes reference to 11 papers in the journal, *Public Library of Science Medicine*, in which experts from the UK and the USA argue that the 'corporate-sponsored creation of disease' is harmful, both to people who may start taking medication as a result, and because it wastes scarce health resources. In case you may have missed the point, the researchers also point out that those who are responsible for defining new diseases are often funded by the drug industry – after identifying a new 'disorder', they can then offer the means to treat it.

If we can accept a situation in which people who are perfectly well can be medicated because they are not feeling as good as they think they ought to be, or because there is some profit to be made, what next? Are we starting to see the beginning of a brave new world of prescribing in which the 'we can fix it' attitude will provide us with a drug for every eventuality? Isn't this the stuff of science fiction? (*see* Box 10.3).

BOX 10.3 Equilibrium

Kurt Wimmer wrote and directed this successful science-fiction film, which was released in 2002, starring Christian Bale and Sean Bean. It is the story of a repressive, fascist regime that depends on the voluntary mass drugging of society to control what is seen to be at the root of all human conflict – emotion. The result is a stark, inhuman 'utopia.' The story plays on a recurrent sci-fi theme – the essential paradox that the faults that threaten our existence are also the very things that make us human.*

Don't worry, be happy, don't think

The 'don't worry – be happy' culture encourages something else that is far more worrying. In Chapter 5 we looked at our rapidly changing society, in which there is an increasing imperative to live life at top speed and do more and more 'multi-tasking.' This has had a number of consequences, not least for family life. However, there are other consequences which, combined with the media imperative to be happy, have resulted in an outcome that should concern us all. It's not only our children who are not thinking – it's us.

If we were to allow ourselves to think, what would we be thinking about? What are some of the thoughts that we would have about children's mental health?

Most of us don't like social injustice, whatever our political persuasion. If we allowed ourselves to think for a minute or two about some of the connections already made between psychological ill health and social adversity, and if we resisted the

---

* Equilibrium (released on 6 December 2002) was directed by Kurt Wimmer and produced by Jan de Bont and Lucas Foster. It starred Christian Bale, Emily Watson and Sean Bean, and was distributed by Dimension Films.

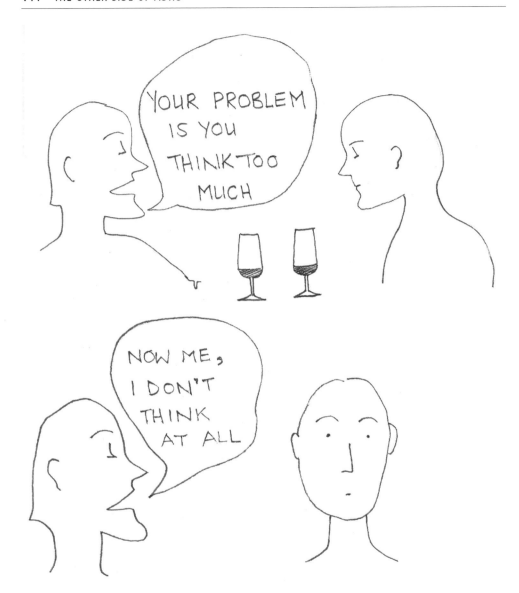

FIGURE 10.1 'The trouble with you . . .'

temptation of the 'Just World' hypothesis that helps us to distance ourselves from the suffering we see around us, we might start thinking about other things, too. We might wonder why it is that these issues never really get addressed. We might ask ourselves why health resources get spent as they do. As Europeans, we might also find ourselves wondering about the pressure on healthcare systems to reform (and in the USA, the pressure not to). We might ask ourselves how all of these things fit into the debate about children's health and well-being and, in particular, the issue of 'ADHD.'

Where do politics come into it?

Politicians can be quite specific in promising 'social change' (whatever that might mean), while many claim to be able to bring 'social justice' (ditto). However, rarely is the rhetoric matched by any real change in the social status quo. One of the key measures of this is inequality in the distribution of healthcare. In the UK, a small flicker of hope that this would begin to change was ignited by the Labour Party election victory in 1997.

One of the first actions of the incoming Labour Party was the commissioning of the Independent Inquiry into Inequalities in Health Report, also known as the Acheson Inquiry, that was published at the end of 1998. Its introduction saw Sir Donald Acheson setting out the remit of the inquiry, in which he stated:

> This report addresses an issue which is fundamentally a matter of social justice, namely that although the last 20 years have brought a marked increase in prosperity and substantial reductions in mortality to the people of this country as a whole, the gap in health between those at the top and bottom of the social scale has widened.[7]

So far, so good, you might think.

This report was to act as a springboard for the government's Action Plan. And what were the results? A subsequent Department of Health commissioned report found that the government had made no inroads into health inequalities at all. In fact, things had got worse. In the years between the commissioning of the original report in 1997 and the data collection in 2001–3, the gap in life expectancy between the bottom fifth and the rest of the population had widened by 21% for males and 51% for females. The poor could still expect to die 7–8 years younger than people living in the wealthiest areas. The infant mortality gap had also continued to widen (from 13% in 1997–9 to 19% in 2001–3).[8]

What happened?

Professor Danny Dorling, a health inequalities expert at Sheffield University, commenting on the failure to address health inequality, noted that 'this is the first Labour Government that has failed to narrow the gap. It is astonishing that after 8 years and making reducing health inequalities a key target that we are in this position.'[9] Dorling has his own explanation for the government's failure: 'Without tackling wealth inequalities, which are widening, it is not going to be able to tackle health inequalities.' And the government's response? There was no sign of them tackling inequalities of wealth. In fact, there was no sign of them tackling any inequalities. Instead, some communities are to be allocated local personalised 'health trainers' to advise us on how to stay healthy. More evidence, you might say, of treating the 'symptoms' rather than the underlying problems.

Of course, this is exactly what politicians are famous for all over the world. Whatever their promises before they come to power, and some might say, their intentions, maintaining themselves in a position of power means that radical change cannot be undertaken without upsetting the rich and powerful, *who are responsible for keeping them in power*. It's a classic political trap. And it is one that makes politicians act not in the interests of the public, whom they are supposed to serve, but in the interests of those who really have the power. If they want to stay in power (and they usually do), their job becomes one of making their decisions seem acceptable to the general public. They become brokers between the real holders of power and the people. They exist to make the unpalatable palatable.

Herein lies the problem. The very act of making 'the unacceptable' attractive enough to make the voters want to vote for you ensures that nothing really changes at all – it is only cosmetically enhanced. The job becomes one of tinkering around the edges to make things acceptable. Reform, rather than revolution, becomes the order of the day. No doubt some readers are thinking to themselves at this point that this is a very good thing – they never voted for revolution anyway. But they *have* collectively voted for change on numerous occasions and have not got it. Now they know why.

Yet there have been substantial changes that I would guess most readers can't remember voting for, but nevertheless have already been initiated. Read on.

Public-sector reform

The public-sector services – health, education and social care – have been subjected to a considerable process of change since the Labour government came to power. It began with the 'modernisation' process, which saw the development of national core standards for local implementation. The modernisation process paved the way for public-sector services that could operate independently from government. The vision for Blair's Britain was one in which the State would no longer be a provider of services. Its role would be to regulate and commission, not just from the public sector but also from private and voluntary agencies. The reality of this new emphasis on public and voluntary 'partnering' is that many public-sector teams, however innovative and successful they might be, find themselves unable to access funding streams that are effectively closed to them, as the 'business' is being directed elsewhere. If this sounds like back-door privatisation, that's because it is.

This advertisement offered additional information to would-be applicants, on request, which stipulated that candidates needed to have experience of managing health budgets of over £300 million. Sam Lister, for *The Times*, informs readers that this means that only the biggest insurers, such as United Healthcare and Kaiser Permanente (both based in the USA), are eligible to apply.

In wide-sweeping reforms spanning health, education, social care, housing, employment, and prison and probation services, markets have been steadily (and stealthily) introduced into the public sector. In keeping with the capitalist ethos, competition between providers is seen as one of the main drivers for cost-effectiveness of treatments, efficiency and quality, all of which, so the theory goes, will be responsive to the demands of the market and offer a greater degree of choice. (Never mind that there is no evidence to support the myth that competition ensures value for money.) As for responsiveness and choice, research also tells us something about this. It tells us that people do not want more choice, they simply want good treatment at their local health facility.

THE TIMES   JUNE 30, 2006

Stealth plan to 'privatise' NHS care
By Sam Lister, Health Correspondent

Health firms to provide 'expert help' and tender for contracts worth billions

The world's biggest private health companies are being invited to bid for the chance to spend substantial chunks of the £80 billion NHS budget.

A six-page 'contract notice' placed by the Department of Health in the supplement to the *Official Journal of the European Union*, and seen by *The Times*, encourages the private sector to apply for a wide range of roles in the control and running of primary care trusts (PCTs).

The trusts are responsible for about 80% of the annual £80 billion NHS budget. They not only fund GP surgeries but also commission hospital operations and have a large say over which drugs patients in their area can receive.

Critics said that the move was like 'putting the NHS up for sale', while some also said it signalled the end of the PCTs' role as providers of clinical services.

Last night, after being contacted by *The Times*, the department suddenly withdrew the advertisement. It said that drafting errors in the document had given the 'false impression' that clinical services provide by PCTs would be phased out in favour of the private sector. However, it insisted that plans to broaden use of 'expert help' from the private sector for ailing PCTs remained accurate.

So what on earth is this all about? What's happening to healthcare? And how does this affect our children?

The changes facing UK citizens are echoed throughout the European Union (EU). Meri Koivusalo, a senior researcher with STAKES,* has warned that the European social model of healthcare provision is under threat. She claims that rapid changes in European health policies have been 'more influenced by internal markets and industrial concerns than by health arguments.' According to Koivusalo, current processes threaten to take European health down the same road as the USA, towards the commercialisation of health systems and away from the social model, out of which has developed the welfare state.[10]

Users of the NHS in the UK have become well used to successive politicians telling them that things in the health service have to change. And they are not stupid. They understand that healthcare has to be affordable, achievable and sustainable. They also understand that if something 'isn't working', there is good justification for change. And this leads us to the following question . . .

---

* STAKES is a Finland-based National Research and Development Centre for Welfare and Health, promoting the welfare and health of the population and developing social and health services.

Does the social model work?

There is widespread support in EU countries for the European healthcare systems. Koivusalo argues that this support is further strengthened by OECD (Organization of Economic Cooperation and Development) data, which show that public healthcare costs are lower in Europe than in the USA. Where rising healthcare costs are concerned, OECD data suggest that they are strongly influenced by two factors, namely the high costs of pharmaceuticals and healthcare technology. It could be argued that both of these factors are eminently alterable, but the types of partnerships that are being forged would seem to militate against this. As Koivusalo is quick to remind us, the drug industry is one of the strongest lobbying forces in the EU, and has been actively represented at a number of levels. As a result there is, as she puts it, a risk of 'inappropriate influence in the name of partnerships.' She writes:

> It is of crucial importance that the EU health strategy does not become a one-stop shop for the pharmaceutical industry and a source for ensuring that member states will invest ever more in pharmaceuticals and health technologies, which form the most rapidly rising part of healthcare costs. This is also crucial when public–private partnerships are addressed.

Advantage or disadvantage?

Whenever public services are opened up to market forces, it seems that it is the more socially disadvantaged who suffer. The more market-driven health systems are, the greater the total healthcare costs and the greater the degree of inequality of access.[11] For Koivusalo, the disadvantages are clear (and would seem to make a mockery of the current emphasis on 'choice'): 'commercialisation of healthcare is not a choice of better off countries but an affliction of the poor.' Box 10.4 summarises the main points behind her argument.

BOX 10.4 Koivusalo's six points about commercialisation and healthcare systems

1 Countries with better health outcomes have significantly lower commercialism of health expenditure.
2 Countries that spend more of their GDP on private health expenditure do not display better outcomes.
3 However, countries that spend more of their GDP on health through public expenditure or social health insurance *do* have significantly better health outcomes.
4 Better care at birth is associated with more of GDP being spent by government or social insurance funds on healthcare, but not with more private healthcare spending.
5 Higher primary care commercialism is associated with greater exclusion of children from treatment when ill.
6 Commercialisation of primary healthcare is associated with greater inequality in rates of consultation for children who are ill.

Given the lack of evidence, you might be forgiven for wondering why there seems to be so much pressure for change.

Koivusalo suggests that some of the pressure is inevitably due to the fact that public budgets are limited. (We need to remember that their limitations are determined by how our governments choose to prioritise.) In addition, public-sector reforms have given added impetus to the growing importance of healthcare as a commercial arena, the further development of which is the business of a range of stakeholders, from 'think tanks', services industries, policy networks and the pharmaceutical industry to international organisations, including the World Bank.

It is noticeable that there has been a change in political rhetoric in line with these developments. This is most evident in the shift in emphasis from capacity issues to the need to diversify and offer 'customer choice.'

Creeping commercialism

Despite a lack of evidence that there are advantages (and mounting evidence that there are disadvantages), the government has been keen to embark on a wave of privately financed health initiatives to build hospitals and clinics and to provide healthcare support services. These are known as Public–Private Partnerships (PPP). The most frequently used PPP is the Private Finance Initiative (PFI). This is essentially a 'rent now, pay later' scheme that can leave authorities struggling to pay large debts as PFI contractors 'refinance' their loans (by this they mean that they change the terms of the loans to increase profits, some by as much as 80%).

At the beginning of 2004, at least 10 NHS hospitals that had been built with private-sector funds were facing debts amounting to £40 million. These debts have continued to rise. Unfortunately, they mask the considerable achievements made by some trusts. For example, the accountants' report for the Audit Commission on the Queen Elizabeth Hospital in Greenwich predicted a £20 million deficit in 2005–6, despite having achieved efficiency levels above the national average. *Half* of this deficit resulted from PFI costs.[12] As another example, consider what has happened to St Bartholomew's and London Trust's PFI project, *the additional cost of which will be over £48 million*. Analysis of eight other PFI schemes shows an increase in annual costs from an average of 4.5% to 16%, once the PFI projects had been completed.[13] Mental health services are particularly vulnerable. One trust in Hertfordshire, forced to make savings of 5%, has cut a range of mental health services, including psychology services.[14]

Another similar initiative to the PFI is the Local Improvement Finance Trust (LIFT), which finances primary care services using private-sector monies. At the time of writing, LIFT schemes have been set up in 26 out of 28 English Strategic Health Authority areas. The model is in the process of being extended to other public services, such as schools. An analysis of the LIFT model has been undertaken by Rachel Aldred at Goldsmiths College, University of London, on behalf of UNISON, the union for public-sector workers. In her report, Aldred analysed six key reasons why LIFT may be a bad deal for the NHS, its customers and those who work within it, as well as for taxpayers.[15] She concluded that the scheme risked putting profit before healthcare needs, was inflexible (owing to the needs of private-sector companies to ensure their cash flow), and presented a conflict of interest, through public–private partnerships that have both investment and regulatory responsibilities. It certainly doesn't seem to represent value for money – the Public Accounts Committee heard that in one area LIFT buildings cost four times more per patient than the average for that area.

There are further concerns that the LIFT schemes will lead to an outsourcing of NHS jobs. This is important in terms of the total care 'package' of the customer, and is a particular concern of UNISON.

UNISON has published several papers on PPPs, and has reached the following conclusion: *'All our evidence and experience shows that once services are run for private profit, the quality of care is reduced and the public-sector ethos is replaced by a hard-nosed profit motive'* (my italics).

Criticism of PPPs is widespread and has arisen from a variety of sources – some unexpected. For instance, Reform, the influential 'non-party' think tank, is a strong force for what it terms 'liberalising' the public sector. Even though it supports the government's general direction of travel, it, too, has called on the NHS to suspend hospital-building programmes using PFI agreements.[16]

Why is the health service in financial difficulty?

Research from Reform provides a breakdown of some of the £3.6 billion invested in English and Welsh hospitals between 2005 and 2006.

£1.8 billion	Pay rises already agreed regarding new consultant contracts, doctors and dentists (*see* Box 10.5 below)
£400 million	New drugs
£320 million	PFI deals
£300 million	Computers
£150 million	Pensions indexation

And what is the change, they ask? 'Zero.'

Consultant contracts

There has been much media discussion of the NHS pay review process known as *Agenda for Change*, a process that has examined and re-banded every single category of NHS job role across the country according to a single pay system. This has proved much more costly than was originally envisaged. Medical consultants have been exempt from this course of action, however, and they have had their contracts negotiated separately, along with GPs (*see* Box 10.5).

Although they have been the subject of considerable criticism, the new consultant contracts are not responsible for the NHS financial crisis. It seems that there are any number of examples of financial 'management' that simply don't make sense. Just a couple of examples of these are given below.

BOX 10.5 The new consultant contracts in the UK health service*

Hospital consultants have been given significant pay rises in return for stricter controls over working practices. Their previous contracts had been 'notoriously preferential.' Bevan described how he had dealt with consultant opposition to the NHS by 'stuffing their mouths with gold.' Since the birth of the NHS, medical consultants have received an NHS salary alongside the right to private practice in NHS beds. They also operated a bonus system that was awarded by consultants, in secret, to each other. The private beds maintained a two-tier system within the health service, while also enabling some consultants to artificially lengthen waiting lists so as to ensure that there was a demand for their private work. Medical consultants became 'the health service's wealthiest, most powerful and least accountable group.' Previous governments had tried, but failed, to make headway with renegotiation of these contracts, and had consistently failed to make medical consultants more accountable for their time.

The current contracts have been negotiated after nearly two years of talks between the BMA and the Department of Health. They provide an increase in 'basic' salary for consultants (up to £85,000) plus extra for other duties, and a maximum working week of 40 hours. Consultants are still entitled to engage in private practice, but no longer during their NHS time. NHS patients are supposed to come first. Medical consultants can earn anything up to around £250,000 from private practice.

The cost of 'management consultants'

Management consultants in the NHS were unheard of until recently. Now it seems that they are everywhere. They are extremely expensive resources. In his speech at the BMA Consultants' Conference in 2006, Paul Miller, Chairman of the Consultants' Committee, provided examples of the ways in which management consultants were currently being used. The first of these was Surrey and Sussex Trust, which during February and March 2005 paid over £52,000 for *less than 2 months* of an interim Chief Executive from a management consultancy firm. Already in difficulty, the trust then brought in more management consultants for half a million pounds.[17]

Miller also criticised the government's keenness on so-called 'Turnaround Teams' from management consultancies. A total of 18 trusts deployed these during 2005–6 at a cost of £100,000 per month in Leeds (£800,000 in total) and £700,000 for 3 months in Surrey and Sussex. (Despite this action, Surrey and Sussex ended 2005–6 with an accumulated deficit of over £57 million. Presumably they didn't ask for a refund after not having been successfully 'turned around.'[18])

The explicit charge throughout Miller's speech was that NHS money was being thrown around haphazardly. This includes the ways in which some executive directors are paid. He draws attention to the fact that the annual report of one trust shows that it paid its executive directors £1.2 million. He also raises the issue of rewarding poor performance, citing as an example the case of the chief executive of one NHS trust in

---

* This information is sourced from *Q+A: the consultant contract* at Guardian.co.uk. Available at http://society. guardian.co.uk/NHSstaff/story/0,,736559,00.html

North-West England, who left after being given a critical external report, yet received a £475,000 pay-off.[19]

Independent-sector treatment centres

The government announced its intention to develop Independent Treatment Centres (ITCs) in 2002. These were to be established as part of its initiative to cut waiting lists by offering non-urgent surgery and diagnostic procedures for NHS patients in privately run centres. The centres were to have their primary areas of focus in medical specialties traditionally associated with long waiting lists, such as orthopaedics and ophthalmology. The first ITCs opened in October 2004. These treatment centres are run by multinational companies with contracts worth billions of pounds. Although they are negotiated nationally, these contracts are paid for locally, a process that creates considerable problems for local commissioners. Many PCTs and hospital trusts have complained that ITCs offer poor value for money and that they divert money away from other services. There have also been concerns about the quality of work undertaken at the centres, with claims of 'botched' operations (*see* Box 10.6) and poor clinical standards.

> ### BOX 10.6 Britain's botched operations – summary by Keep our NHS Public[20]
>
> A BBC investigation has uncovered an alarmingly high number of botched operations by foreign surgeons working in private treatment centres for the NHS. One confidential health authority audit of 70 operations at a private hospital found 'serious concerns' about 67% of them. David Dandy, Vice-President of the Royal College of Surgeons, said: 'in 40 years experience, I have never come across quite so many operations needing to be repeated in such a short time.' For example, of 18 operations carried out by Arpad Illyes from Hungary, 12 were found by an independent surgeon to be poor. For another doctor, Roland Istria, of 15 operations, nine were found to be poor – a failure rate of 66%. The average NHS failure rate in the field is 2%. There is concern about statistics, most of which the government will not release due to commercial confidentiality. In the case of one botched hip replacement, because corrective surgery was later carried out by the NHS, the procedure was recorded as an overall success.

A number of critics have suggested that ITCs are wasteful of NHS resources. In some areas – for example, Oxfordshire and Nottinghamshire – ITCs have resulted in NHS facilities lying idle.[21] The government has been accused of setting up facilities that are not needed, with contracts having to be paid for whether they are used or not. For instance, in the case of Greater Manchester, £1.9 million was paid to Netcare for operations that were not performed, as patients opted for NHS procedures instead. The ITC performed 2,000 fewer operations than anticipated, but the contract between the PCTs and Netcare meant that the full amount had to be paid. This arrangement alone meant a loss to the NHS of almost £2 million pounds over a 6-month period. These are not isolated examples – the pattern is repeated across the country. You might wonder what the government's response has been. With disheartening predictability it has been, of course, to extend the ITC programme.

Paul Miller, speaking at the annual BMA Consultants' Conference, had this to say:

> If you had made this up, you would be laughed at.
>
> If you were the one who did make this up, you should be ashamed.
>
> If you continue to make it happen, you will destroy our NHS.
>
> This is not the way to run the NHS.
>
> Care is suffering, jobs are disappearing, patients and staff are paying the price.

Some might feel that the spectacle of Miller's consultants and those responsible for ITCs, inefficiency 'pay-offs' and other damaging initiatives wagging their fingers at each other smacks of rather too much irony – they are all part of the same culture. Nevertheless, it is hard not to agree with Miller's point that 'the emperor of English health policy is wearing no clothes.'

The ongoing saga of the NHS IT project

No critique of NHS spending, however brief, can avoid mentioning the disaster that has been the NHS National Programme for Information Technology (NPfIT). This project has been beset by problems since it was first announced in June 2002. There has been a series of delays and missed deadlines, coupled with progress that has been so problematic that some trusts have abandoned their involvement in it and are seeking alternative solutions. The project was originally costed at £2.3 billion, but is already massively over budget. It has been suggested that the final cost could be as high as £30 billion, a figure that is more than 10 times the original estimate and represents 30 times the current deficit in the NHS.[22]

This is a continuation of a long series of disastrous information projects in the NHS, many of which have been abandoned after millions of pounds have been, effectively, poured down the drain. One high-profile example is the Wessex Regional Health Authority Information Systems Plan (RISP), which was abandoned in 1990 after more than £43 million had been spent. Another such example is the London Ambulance Service Computer-Aided Despatch (LASCAD) project, which was dropped after it had already cost £7.5 million. A year later, a further attempt was made to provide this system, which also failed.[23] These two cases received a great deal of publicity, unlike later examples such as the Hospital Information Support Systems (in 1997) and the Clinical Coding Information System (in 1998), both of which failed, at enormous cost to the NHS.

What's the problem with the NHS?

Ask anyone who works in the health service what the difficulties are and they will be able to tell you. NHS workers have endured years of constant reform, deconstruction and reorganisation, with the result that they are stressed, demotivated and defeated by this. They want to do their jobs, and most of them are extremely dedicated and have made a deliberate choice to work in the health service. But they will tell you that it has become increasingly difficult – if not impossible – to do their work. One of the main problems is over-management (despite government assertions that the opposite is the case), leading to the majority of the working week being spent in 'business' meetings (which require some preparatory work) or providing vast amounts of information for various departments within the organisation. Many will tell you that there is less clinical work going on than there has ever been. The target-driven culture of recent years has led to a mushrooming of management of nuclear explosion proportions, and has given rise to hundreds of departments, services and teams, whose task is to produce reports, strategies or plans that demonstrate progress. This process ends up driving itself. And what is the product? Glossy strategies that can't be delivered because there aren't enough staff. More targets. More teams to help us to achieve them. It can all start to sound, well, a little déjà vu.

BOX 10.7 Recognise this?[*]

We trained hard, but it seemed every time we were beginning to form up into teams, we would be reorganised. I was to learn later in life that we tend to meet any new situation by reorganising, and a wonderful method it can be for creating the illusion of progress while producing confusion, inefficiency and demoralisation.

From Petronii Arbitri Satyricon, AD 66 (attributed to Gaius Petronus, a Roman general who later committed suicide)

For many, the problem lies in the continuing drive towards commercialism (and the focus on this at the expense of other priorities), coupled with the failure of the decision makers to appreciate the important differences between a *business* and a *service*.

Despite their fatigue and low morale, those same workers who are able to tell you what is wrong with the NHS will also be able to tell you what is right. And they would say that there is a great deal right. Their worries are that the baby is about to be thrown out with the bath water.

What's the solution?

Paul Miller's BMA speech included a number of comments about what characteristics 'his' kind of NHS would have. My guess is that most of these would tally with the rest of the owners of the NHS (that means you and me, by the way).

---

[*] I am grateful to Jon Courthold, Clinical Psychologist with North Staffordshire Combined Healthcare Trust, for sending this quotation to fellow psychologists and psychological therapists working in the NHS.

- The NHS I believe in would always remain funded from taxation, free at the point of patient need.
- It would treat patients according to their clinical need, not political targets.
- It would put patients first by aiming to bring all NHS facilities up to scratch, not by offering them a false choice of taking their custom elsewhere.
- It would focus on improving standards of patient care by clinical networks, not on using 'creative destruction' to force 're-management' of 'failing trusts.'
- It would concentrate on good quantitative and qualitative data from IT systems to improve patient care, not just for producing bills.
- It would not be constantly torn apart and turned around by 'initiativitis.'
- It would realise that by respecting staff it will get the best for its patients.
- It would employ good managers for the long term, not for short-term projects or dirty work.
- It would be run at arm's length from politicians, who do not have the ability to run it, or allow it to be run for the best.
- It would put clinical collaboration before commercial competition.
- And it would always put patients before profits.[24]

Although I don't personally agree with Miller's solution, which is to effectively put the medical consultants back in charge, I think he has made a good start with this list. His only mistake, for me, is to suggest that there needs to be a greater distance between the health service and 'the politicians.' Given the history of the past 25 years, many might feel instead that the problems only really began in earnest when we tried to pretend that political beliefs and actions could be separated from real life and, for the present purposes, from healthcare responsibility and decision making.

What has all of this got to do with ADHD?

ADHD has been a phenomenon of proportions we have simply never seen before anywhere in the world. An unprecedented number of children are being labelled and medicated as a result, many of whom are living in adverse social circumstances that in themselves are enough to explain their difficulties, without the need to resort to medical 'diagnoses.' In choosing to view children's difficulties as 'disorders', rather than as the result of what we as adults do to them, we collude with a system that invites us to adopt an attitude of passivity and indifference. ADHD is a phenomenon that involves all of these processes. It is also a reflection of how we think about and treat children in our society. Most of all, the evidence suggests that the epidemic of ADHD is a direct result of increasingly close partnerships with drug companies. And the signs are that there is more to come.

For example, in a recent visit to one of Staffordshire's hospitals, Lord Warner, Minister for State in charge of health reforms, cited *as an example of progress* a new local state-of-the-art primary care centre that had been set up in partnership with one of the drug companies. This drug company was also providing training for the staff. It is worrying that Lord Warner seemed to be unaware of the potential conflict of interest in such a venture, and the ensuing risk that it poses to patients. Instead, he chose to trumpet it as *the new way of working.**

This 'new approach' to healthcare threatens to open up mental health to the worst possible kind of rampant market forces, while offering service users titbits that look attractive and suggest improvements and increased accessibility: 'Won't it be nice for you all when you have an opportunity to pay a quick visit to a GP when you happen to be in Boots the Chemist?' Well, no, actually – this is pretty meaningless trivia if it means that the whole of the healthcare infrastructure is being systematically wrecked and shipped off to the scrapyard at the same time.

Legitimising these decidedly dubious partnerships strengthens the biological psychiatry model, on which they depend. In order to be worth doing, from the drug companies' point of view, there must be profits to be made, and this can only mean more drugs (and more 'disorders' to be 'treated'). While we invest in drug treatment, other approaches to mental health – and this includes 'ADHD' – will continue to be poorly resourced, scare and difficult to obtain. Ask yourself the following questions. Are partnerships with drug companies likely to lead to more or less prescribing? In whose interests are these 'partnerships'? Are they really in the interests of your child?

As we move towards greater commercialisation of healthcare systems in Europe, the future looks neither bright nor orange – it looks American. And although it seems entirely reasonable to study (and learn from) other healthcare systems in other countries, it looks as if it is the USA that is emerging as the model for developing social and health policies. Indeed, Lord Warner seemed delighted to tell his audience in Staffordshire that he had just returned from the USA, where he had been looking at the Medicare/Medicaid system. The fact that the US system seems to be acting as a template for UK services, despite its obvious weaknesses, is viewed by many to be strongly linked to economic and business interests. It seems likely that both governments have already set off down a pathway that remains deliberately obscured from the public gaze. The kinds of developments and initiatives that are already in process have not been opened up for public debate at all, nor are they part of the Labour Party's manifesto. (For a comparison of extracts from the 1997 Labour Party Manifesto and the position and plans in 2006, *see* Appendix 2.)

ADHD is the first so-called 'disorder' of its kind that I can recall since beginning my career in psychology many years ago. It is the first 'new' problem that I can remember being identified during all this time, and certainly the only one I can remember – ever – that was claimed, from the start, to be neurobiological and to require drug treatment. ADHD may be the 'first wave' of a new approach to children's mental health – an approach that accepts as legitimate the drugging of children who have no identifiable mental disorder. If we allow this situation to continue, what will be next? What other 'disorders' will follow? How shall we ever get the kind of focus that is needed on the real issues in children's lives that affect their physical and psychological well-being? All of these issues make ADHD an intensely political issue.

---

* Staff question-and-answer session during Lord Warner's visit to South Staffordshire Healthcare NHS Foundation Trust on 29 July 2006.

It is important that we are all able to think about these things, however difficult and unpleasant they may be. While we are sleep-walking through life, things are happening. Soon it will be too late.

CHAPTER 11

Where do we go from here?

The drug companies have a huge vested interest in continuing to promote ADHD as a 'real' diagnostic category, a biological brain disorder that should be treated with drugs (theirs, of course). Despite decades of substantial worldwide investment in research that has failed to provide any robust evidence either that ADHD is a biological brain disorder or that it has a genetic basis, the message from the pro-ADHD lobby remains the same. The evidence is 'developing', they say. But how long must we continue to 'treat' children while we wait for this evidence to 'develop'? Another 25 years? In the search for ADHD 'proof', a large body of information has amassed, including real-life stories about real children who deserve better than this. We have learned that the side-effects of stimulant medication for children are more serious than was first thought. This, together with concerns about the longer-term impact on the developing brain, makes the 'cure' not only worse than the 'complaint' but, frankly, not worth the risk.

We embarked on this route more than a quarter of a century ago, without any knowledge of what we were really doing to children or why. But it was done anyway. All this time we have continued to monitor, to engage in further studies and to add to our 'theories' of what might be happening. The fact that we have effectively used children in this way, as part of some vast clinical trial, should provoke international outrage. Many children have suffered as a result, and some have died. The evidence suggests that this issue has not been driven by health concerns, or even by science, but by profit.

The more you look at the research and clinical evidence, the less likely it seems that what is described as ADHD is any kind of unitary trait at all. At most, it seems to be a diagnostic label that lumps together some fairly common childhood characteristics, the desirability of which depends, inevitably, on how they are socially constructed. They can, it seems, include 'symptoms' that lie on the periphery of other problems, such as attachment difficulties, chronic stress or trauma, as well as including a fair few correlates of general childhood distress. The economic and social disadvantages that have been shown to map on to children's so-called 'mental health disorders' should call into question for all of us the validity of such a system for classifying children's problems – or anyone else's, for that matter.

A number of writers have suggested that 'ADHD' is a good descriptor for children who have not got the attention they need from adults. (This means all of us, by the way, not just parents. It refers to teachers, doctors, mental health practitioners, social workers, police, members of the public and government ministers, to name but a few.) Knowing, as we do, that the children and young people – mostly boys – who receive this diagnosis are likely to be those who have to cope with the worst that life can throw at them, how can we justify using a biological label to describe the psychological distress that ensues? Shame on all of us.

ADHD has become a diagnostic 'peg' on which to hang everything, especially those things we don't know what to do with because they don't seem to fit anywhere else. This represents a serious mislabelling of the difficulties that young people have, and therefore translates as an unforgivable failure to provide them with the help that they need. Their problems are not ameliorated by pharmacology – they are merely blunted by it. If anyone seriously believes that this is an 'improvement', they are deluding themselves.

Children continue to be the silent minority for whom very few people speak. They are at the mercy of adults who make their healthcare decisions. They are seldom asked for their consent to treatment, but they are treated anyway. The UK House of Commons Health Committee inquiry into the influence of the pharmaceutical industry made mention of children only four times in about 550 pages of oral and written submissions. Even then, they were brief references that were not developed. This is not unusual. It is rare to find any meaningful focus on children in discussions about mental health issues, unless it is in a specific children's forum. Thus our most vulnerable group remains outside people's thinking on issues that are critical to their human rights. This is reflected in services, where, for many years, children's mental health was known as one of the 'Cinderella services', due to funding disparities between children's and adult services. Despite promised funding increases to improve child and adolescent mental health provision, differences remain and when 'mental health' is under discussion, there continues to be an assumption that we are talking about adults. Only a system such as this, which does not attach a high priority to children, and where children have no voice and no representation, could allow such a swift and successful under-the-radar development and colonisation of 'ADHD.' Only a political system that considers greed to be an acceptable trait could sanction the existing practices of the drug companies and those who collude with them in perpetuating 'ADHD' as a 'disorder' that necessitates children being drugged in vast numbers.

Why we need biological explanations

We have dug ourselves into a hole. Most parents and mental health professionals know that when children do this, it's time to think creatively of ways to help them to get out again without their having to lose face in the process. It's difficult to know how the medical establishment and the government – both of which are in cahoots with the drug industry – can do this. As Peter Breggin has written, the biological psychiatrists are in a position where to admit that mental health difficulties are not biological threatens their very existence. After all, why have medics in the first place if problems are not medical? And it follows that if these difficulties are not medical, pharmacological solutions would make no sense. We are well and truly stuck in the hole. The only solution, it seems, is to keep digging, maintaining a precarious 'bit of both' balance. This position maintains the current status quo while being precarious enough to make it a taboo subject in the multi-disciplinary mental health arena. We self-censor.[1] We seek compromise where really we should seek to challenge.

Why we need the drug companies

The pharmaceutical industry is seen as one of the strengths of the UK economy. In 2003, £3.5 billion were invested by the drug companies in research and development in the UK. This represents a quarter of all research and development in the UK. The industry was also responsible for about £11.8 billion in exports, resulting in a trade surplus of over £3 billion. Sales of UK pharmaceuticals come to nearly £9 billion (these are all 2001 figures). A total of 69,000 people are employed directly by the industry, and a further 25,000 are employed in related industries. The drug companies are the largest employers of science graduates in the country. One-third of the UK-based industry is UK owned and one-third is US owned.[2]

The government plan is to extend the research base, which includes the NHS, through close working with the companies, thus attracting more business and investment. This is a key component of their planning for the UK economy. The drug industry is therefore a key element in economic growth, as it is in the rest of Europe, and is looking for a 'supportive regulatory environment.' It is not averse to using its financial muscle to try to achieve this. For example, the pharmaceutical giant Pfizer recently made its impatience with the UK planning system known when it abandoned a plan to locate its European headquarters in Surrey, and instead moved to Germany, where the regulatory environment is more relaxed.[3] This will have come as a huge blow to the UK which, you can bet, will have received the intended message. Just a week later the Chancellor of the Exchequer, Gordon Brown, announced that he had embarked on a 'streamlining' of planning rules, following concerns that the UK was failing to respond to international competition.[4] One of the effects of 'relaxing' regulations so that they favour big business is that they also make it easier for large-scale, possibly contentious plans to be fast-tracked, with much less consultation.

The 'business climate' in the UK will be increasingly important in determining its attractiveness to international investment. This means more pressure for deregulation and the development of favourable business environments in order to compete in the global market. After all, globalisation means giving priority to corporate interests, however much the pro-globalisation contingent might like to think otherwise.

The bioscience plan

What's the plan for the UK? One of the key elements of the plan is undoubtedly bioscience development, which has been referred to as the 'jewel in the crown' in terms of future economic development (and a key element of this is pharmaceuticals). No secret has been made of the importance of the NHS to this process of making the country 'a very attractive place for business to come and operate.'[5] The government is therefore entangled in its own conflict of interest. Its economic plan for the country relies on bioscience being at its epicentre, which means that it needs industries integral to that to grow and develop. It cannot encourage these developments while at the same time adequately protecting its citizens. This is illustrated by the current NICE guidelines fiasco in which the government seems to think it is perfectly acceptable for the drug companies to be involved in drawing up the policies of the NHS, to which it then sells the drugs that those policies recommend. No amount of rhetoric can make sense of these kinds of practices. The lack of acknowledgement by the government of the inappropriateness of such an arrangement and the danger that it poses to NHS users is shocking. It also brings to life the famous definition of politics made by the philosopher and educator John Dewey, as 'the shadow cast on society by big business.'[6]

The pharmaceutical industry knows full well how important it is in this process. One of the stated aims of the American Pharmaceutical Group (APG) is to 'advise how the UK can attract inward investment from the US.' Inevitably, they see the blurring of public and private sectors as 'creating more opportunities.' They are clear how much the UK needs the APG to turn it into a market leader. In its submission to the House of Commons Committee, the drug company Novartis, which makes Ritalin, has a subtitle that reads, 'Contribution to UK plc.' (Novartis spends £50 million per year on research and development in the UK.)

The APG submission to the same investigation includes the statement (repeated verbatim) in Box 11.1.

BOX 11.1 Low utilisation of new medicines

There are specific areas of concern in the UK. Out of 10 comparator developed countries . . . the UK had the lowest take-up of new medicines launched within the last 5 years, and the proportion is falling. On current trends, the UK has already been or soon will be overtaken by Japan, the only country with a worse record, so UK patients will receive more dated medicines than any other comparator country.

One aspect (but only one aspect) of this poor take-up is the persistence of postcode prescribing across the NHS, although NICE was established in part to eliminate this. All patients should have the right to know about the best medicines that are available and to receive them, so that postcode prescribing is eliminated.

I would like to repeat this APG submission, together with my own subtext for interested readers.

Low utilisation of new medicines

There are specific areas of concern in the UK. Out of 10 comparator developed
We are particularly worried about your failure to completely buy into our propaganda in the UK.

countries . . . the UK had the lowest take-up of new medicines launched within the
*In all other European countries where we have aggressively marketed our products over the
last 5*

last 5 years, and the proportion is falling. On current trends, the UK has already
been
*years, there has been a good take-up of new products, but not you. Just the opposite. If you
continue*

or soon will be overtaken by Japan, the only country with a worse record,
*to make your own reasoned judgements about these things, you'll stand out as one of the
only*

so UK patients will receive more dated medicines than any other
*countries that continues to use tried and tested medicines, rather than changing to new ones
in order*

comparator country.
to subsidise our already highly profitable industry, using public monies.

One aspect (but only one aspect) of this poor take-up is the persistence of
*You needn't think that you can just do what you want in relation to your local population.
It's lucky*

postcode prescribing across the NHS, although NICE was established in part to
*for us that we are involved in writing the NICE guidelines that will stop you acting
independently*

eliminate this. All patients should have the right to know about the best
*once and for all. We will then ensure that our propaganda is distributed to all prescribers
and all*

medicines that are available and to receive them, so that postcode prescribing is
patients in the NHS. Then we'll ensure that your patients will want the latest, more
expensive drugs.

eliminated.
You've been warned.

The corporate takeover of learning

In recent years, something unthinkable has happened – science has become questionable.
We now live in times in which the research climate seems to be that anything can be
'proven' according to one's agenda. Information sites have been flooded with pseudo-

research, reported on an almost daily basis in the media and even in respectable scientific journals. With its integrity compromised, research, whose purpose should be to add to the knowledge base, becomes little more than propaganda. This issue was raised during the House of Commons Health Committee's investigation into the influence of the pharmaceutical industry, with Sir Iain Chalmers describing the industry's influence on the scientific record as 'indefensible and sly.'[7] Sir Iain also commented on the 'economic power of the industry' to determine what is studied in the first place. Its influence, he reminded us, is far reaching, extending beyond individual academics to entire institutions.

The agenda of science and technology is being set by the drug industry, within the wider context of big business. The profit agenda determines the nature of our developing knowledge base. This represents the corporate takeover of learning and leads to a situation where *we only learn what can make money for the big corporations*. Taken to its extreme, it means that learning stops altogether. There are some who are concerned that this process has already begun.

Why there should be more of a challenge . . .

It would be as wrong to give the impression that all psychiatrists are supportive of the increasing focus on the biological model as it would be to imply that psychiatrists have been entirely uncritical of the ensuing developments in mental health. Quite a number of them have spoken out. The Critical Psychiatry Network, which was formed in 1999, describes itself as 'sceptical' about the medical model, and disagrees with the emphases that have been placed on biological research and treatment. It states that 'we do not seek to justify psychiatric practice by postulating brain pathology as the basis for mental illness.'[8] In common with other psychiatrists, like Peter Breggin, the network has raised specific concerns about the Mental Health Act, which can compel people to take medication, sometimes for long periods, without their consent. It points out that the extension of this Act in 1983 extends these powers into the community. It cautions that 'This change in the law has major ethical implications. It is absolutely essential that there should be no concerns about the integrity or the factual basis of the evidence for the efficacy and safety of drugs that are likely to be used in this way. All the evidence indicates that this is not the case.'

In an attempt to break up the cosy relationships between doctors and drug companies, the government is using a tried and tested method – paying them to do it differently.

The UK is embarking on what it calls 'direct incentives' for doctors who achieve targets, which the Critical Psychiatry Network believes may be beneficial in motivating them 'to be wary of drug promotion that conflicts with the achievement of quality targets.'

In other words, the NHS will pay them extra, as an alternative to them seeking the additional money from the drug companies. The Critical Psychiatry Network might not be quite removed enough to see the continued irony in the government's approach to doctors. This strategy, like others (for instance, the consultants' new NHS contracts), is based on the idea that you need to outbid the competition to get doctors on side. In a way that (depressingly) acknowledges if not colludes with the corruption and greed inherent in many practices tolerated by the NHS, the suggested deal will pay doctors *not to do the wrong thing*. Would you like to be paid extra incentives for doing your job properly? So would I!

What's in a label?

What does it mean to be an ADHD non-believer? For a start, it doesn't mean that I don't help young people who might have the kind of difficulties that would give them an ADHD label. I do. My approach is to try to find ways to help them and their families to overcome these problems, as I have always done. The label itself, or rather the lack of it, would not affect the approaches I would use as a clinical psychologist (including those I might use to help me to determine whether what I was doing was having any impact on my client's problems). In approaching people's problems in this way, I would not be very different from a great many other psychological therapists and counsellors. Labels, for the most part, are not usually all that helpful to people, unless they need them as a kind of 'passport' to other types of help or to drug treatment (and the need for a 'passport' should in itself be contentious). The reason why they are not helpful is that most people's problems do not fit into nice neat diagnostic boxes – they are unique, just like the people who have them.

The pro-ADHD lobby has a particular attitude towards people like me. Among other things, they accuse us of 'upsetting' the families of children with 'ADHD' and of 'blaming' parents. These are childish and deliberately emotive accusations. They are also untrue. Many of us who have chosen to speak out about this issue are practising clinicians who have substantial experience of day-to-day work with children, young people and families, *and are still doing it*. We are not in the business of giving up on families, and we spend a good portion of our working life advocating for them. We know how hard a job it is to be a parent. We also know that, although there may be any number of things that combine to cause children to be unhappy or anxious, whether these problems get better or worse will often depend on how things are in the family. In other words, whatever the problem, we understand from experience that the family is going to be a significant part of the solution. If anyone sees this as making us 'anti-family', they are completely missing the point.

By way of illustration, I would like to tell you about David. I first met him and his parents when he was 14 years old and had been temporarily excluded from school on the grounds of poor behaviour. David had been adopted by his parents, Bob and Helen, at the age of 8 years. They had two grown-up children, whom they had also adopted, and who now lived independently. They were a close family and David liked to be treated to a weekend away with his oldest brother, who had completed college and lived with his partner. David's birth mother had been in contact with the family some years ago and Helen encouraged this, even facilitating a couple of visits. Nothing came of this relationship, however, and David was left feeling abandoned when his mother disappeared and left him no contact details.

David presented a lot of challenges to his parents, and they had to work hard at times 'just to get through.' Bob and Helen were not only experienced parents, but they were also experienced adopters, who were able to understand how David's past experiences gave meaning to his present behaviours. In family meetings with myself and my colleague, a family therapist, they all made good progress, which showed itself in a number of ways, including improvements in relationships, as well as in David's behaviour. He continued to have some classroom difficulties, such as having problems paying attention, being easily distracted and often being non-compliant. David and I agreed to spend a few sessions together looking at how he could put himself in charge of these behaviours. He made excellent progress (*see* Box 11.2).

BOX 11.2 Paying attention to David

I shared with David some of my ideas about why it was sometimes hard to cope in the classroom. I talked with him about how it is that young people can sometimes get really good at not thinking, and also how their heads can get absolutely full of other things that stop them concentrating on what they should be doing. David wanted some support with these things because he was fed up with getting into trouble. Together we devised a few 'tricks' that might help him. One that he particularly liked involved him self-monitoring in a notebook. He designed the monitoring 'grid' himself and decided on time intervals. He was to put his watch on his desk and give himself a 'tick' for every 10 minutes he remained on task. He and I had a bet about how many ticks he would get per day. Of course he won, and each victory resulted in a small stationery item (he had a full pencil case by the time we finished doing this work). This strategy, and others, would not have worked, of course, without the participation of the school. I gave the school as helpful a description as I could of my involvement with David, and I was careful to include the solution-focused trick of asking them to note down and inform me of any improvements they noticed, given that I couldn't be there all the time in person. I wrote a number of therapeutic letters to David (and a couple to his year tutor). David's letters would include another tip to help him with his attention and motivation, such as how to use self-talk, how to organise himself using a planner, and so on. Just one at a time. The improvement in David's behaviour was noticeable to everyone.

This improvement was not just about David – it was also about his teachers starting to focus on what he was doing right, rather than what he was doing wrong. His parents, too, became more relaxed because they were not being constantly telephoned by David's teachers and they knew he was receiving some special help from me. This is the nature of therapy – a little pebble in the pond can make quite a few ripples.

Valuing children, valuing ourselves

Peter Breggin said in his book, *Toxic Psychiatry*, 'Nothing measures the quality of a society better than how it treats its children.' If he's right, we are in trouble. Authors and clinicians like Sami Timimi have commented on Western society's ambivalence towards children – 'demonising' children appears to be something we became particularly good at as the twentieth century drew to a close. 'ADHD' seems to be a particularly appropriate diagnosis for societies that have less and less time for children. A number of commentators have suggested that 'ADHD' is the re-labelling of ordinary childhood behaviour, making it disordered – as such, it represents the medicalisation of childhood. Some writers, like Thom Hartmann, have suggested that 'ADHD' constitutes a negative reframing of behaviours that can be positive qualities or traits. There are worries that the Ritalin generation will be able to sit still in class but will have lost the ability to be creative.[9]

Making a difference

Sometimes it's difficult to believe that you can make a difference to what's happening. It can seem as if there is just no point in trying to do anything or influence anyone because, in the end, it will be a waste of time – the people who make the decisions will simply go ahead and do what they want anyway. There are people who believe that this attitude is subtly encouraged by those in power.

Much earlier in this book we looked at what has been happening to modern life (and whether, as some people thought, it might indeed be 'rubbish'). In trying to make sense of some of the difficulties that our children are having, it is important to look at the context of their lives, which of course are our lives as well. In a world that is becoming more and more marked by loosening family bonds, conspicuous consumption, multi-tasking and sensory bombardment, it seems understandable that our children, like us, are not paying attention. In such a world, 'attention' is also a means to an end, as the academic and political activist, Noam Chomsky, reminds us when he warns of a public relations industry whose purpose it is to create 'artificial wants' and to focus attention on superficial aspects of life while at the same time cultivating a sense of futility that ensures consumers do not try to take control of their own lives.[10]

In an inspiring call to arms, Chomsky encourages us to challenge the slogan 'There Is No Alternative', which he describes as 'a self-serving fraud.' He adds, 'The particular socio-economic order that's being imposed is the result of human decisions in human institutions. The decisions can be modified; the institutions can be changed. If necessary, they can be dismantled and replaced, just as honest and courageous people have been doing throughout the course of history.'

What is to be done about the drug companies?

This book contains a lot of criticism of the drug companies. It is therefore only fair that I should present some ideas about how things could be different.

Current practices bring medicine into disrepute. It should be obvious by now that self-regulation does not work, and urgent action is needed to restore confidence in doctors. There is much talk about the need for more transparency (as if that will do the trick), but transparency is not enough. This really is an example of 'tinkering at the edges' (remember that?), and it will never be enough. There is a pathology in the system so great that reform will just not do it.

There is an urgent need for the complete uncoupling of the drug industry from medicine, as well as a need for much more rigorous controls, underpinned by legislation that is clear and not open to interpretation. The following are just some suggestions about what could be done for starters.

- *Raising awareness* – we need to start by alerting people to the mistakes that have been made, and being honest about the reasons why change is needed.
- All regulatory bodies should include members of the public.
- Regulation should be independent.
- Membership by those who have any current or past involvement in drug companies should not be permitted.
- Funding of patient groups should be illegal.
- Consultation with patients should be via a network of 'expert patients' who, through their routine courses of treatment, would be able to 'sign up' to acting as a consultant at any time, should they wish to do so.
- There should be no 'direct-to-customer' information – such material should be provided by an independent body, whose explicit function is to be balanced.
- All hospitality and promotional activity should be banned.
- All clinical trials should be registered at the outset.
- All results of such trials should be made public, not just those that the drug companies want us to know about.
- An independent register of adverse reactions should be maintained.
- Research governance should be free from all drug company influence.
- Education and training should be free from all drug industry influence.
- There should be a clear rationale behind the development of any new drug.
- If biotechnologies are to flourish, there is an urgent need for discussion about how profits should be invested, and whether there should be a requirement for a proportion of the profits to be reinvested in healthcare services and in other not-for-profit activities (e.g. in developing countries).
- Breaking the above rules should lead to loss of licence.[*]

This list will no doubt be incomplete, and readers will perhaps come up with their own suggestions as to how the industry can be better regulated. The point is, if you and I and a few others can do it, it is eminently do-able. Some of these points, and others, were made in the House of Commons Health Committee recommendations arising from their inquiry into the influence of the pharmaceutical industry. It will be interesting to see what follows.

What's to be done about ADHD?

When I set out to write this book, I wanted to present to the reader some of the important issues that had brought ADHD into being and were continuing to affect

---

[*] I would like to be able to claim that these are all my own ideas, but they are not. Many of them are gleaned from my reading of the recommendations of others, such as the contributors to the House of Commons Health Committee's inquiry into the influence of the pharmaceutical industry.[2]

thinking about mental health generally. I wanted the reader to understand why it is that ADHD is such a controversial subject, and to understand something about what the controversy was all about. I hoped to make the connections between this controversy and some other, highly contentious developments which have also grown on the back of the bio-psychiatry culture and its incestuous relationship with the pharmaceutical industry. ADHD is not the first of their progeny, but *it is the first of its kind for children*. This, and the kind of judgements that come into play when a child is 'diagnosed', makes it a political diagnosis. For those readers who prefer their health with not so much politics, I apologise. I just can't seem to find a way to do it differently. Above all, I wanted to bring some of the important evidence together that would enable me to tell a story that I felt very strongly needed to be told. This is the story you seldom hear – the 'other side' of the story. So this is an unapologetically one-sided book, presenting, as it does, only one side of the story. If you want the other side, it's easily accessible. It's all around you. This is the end of this one.

The wildest colts make the best horses.
(Themistocles, 525–460 BC)[*]

---

* I hadn't come across this quotation before I read it in Peter Breggin's book, *Toxic Psychiatry*. Now it's one of my favourites.

Looking after our children

Children do not have disorders: they live in a disordered world.
Peter Breggin

What children need

We already know what children need. We know this from a significant body of research, as well as from clinical experience. Children need environmental conditions that support their growth and emotional development, rather than hinder them. These include adequate basic needs (to be safe, warm, clothed, fed and adequately looked after), to live in a home that affords adequate shelter and fulfils health and hygiene needs, to live in conditions that allow access to the outdoors, and a place to play in a neighbourhood that is safe. Children also need lives that are as free as possible from adverse social circumstances, including parental mental ill health, drug and alcohol abuse, violence, physical, emotional and sexual abuse, family breakdown and other traumas. When they do encounter adversity, we know that responsive, loving parents moderate the effects of these traumas, helping to ensure that their children remain emotionally healthy. We already know these things.

In terms of parenting, we know that a child does better with two parents. These parents will make a better job of parenting if they have themselves been loved, valued and well parented. If they haven't, they can still be good parents, but they will need to have worked out their own difficulties and be of sufficient emotional maturity to have made sense of their experiences. If not, they will play out their own unprocessed traumas through their children, perpetuating the cycle.

Parenting is easier if the parents love and value each other. This will be sensed by their children, whether they like it or not. Being loved also makes it possible for the adults to give love. A loving relationship is also one in which conflicts are more likely to be resolved in a healthy way. This in turn provides a good model for children. Pregnancies go better if they are relatively stress-free, and this is another reason why two parents are better than one. The pregnant mother needs to be nurtured so that she can do the nurturing after the baby is born.

We know that children need to develop a secure attachment to a caregiver, and that this is one of the most important determinants of their emotional well-being. This requires carers to be available and responsive.

Pre-school

The child needs the structure of a safe, predictable environment where there are clear limits and boundaries. He or she needs regular mealtimes and good food, of sufficient quantity and quality to facilitate healthy development. The parents need to be united in their management of the child's behaviour. Parents should focus on shaping behaviour by attention and praise (for good behaviour). They should use ignoring and distraction for 'minor' bad behaviour, and consequences for bad behaviour that can't be ignored. Consequences should always be brief and should be followed by completely back-to-normal behaviour. A good daytime routine should be developed, along with a good bedtime and sleep routine. All young children need a regular bedtime, preceded by a wind-down routine, which can include story time. Televisions, VCRs and DVD players in bedrooms are never a good idea for young children. Bed should be a place to sleep, and if this is established early on, it should not be a problem. (If you get the little things right at this stage, you won't have to deal with the bigger things later on.)

School age

When children start school, structure and routine become even more important. Children need help and support with managing the new regime, starting to organise themselves, starting to plan, undertaking any tasks set by the teacher and coping with the social aspects of school. They need help making friends and managing conflict. They also need help managing injustice, when it happens. This is when all the hard work you have put in while helping your child to manage his or her emotions will pay off. If you haven't done this and you have allowed your child to behave like a monster at home, don't be surprised when he or she becomes one at school. If this happens to you, all is not lost, but you will need to go back to parenting basics and join forces with the school. Don't be tempted to collude with your child against the teacher, but instead be prepared to tackle the real problems. (Remember that if you get the little things right at this stage, you won't have to deal with the bigger things later on.)

Adolescence

One of the main tasks of adolescence is for the young person to develop an identity for him- or herself outside the family. During this time, parents need to do a tricky balancing act of maintaining boundaries and limits while also being flexible. They also need to find the balancing point between *preparing* their child for adulthood and *protecting* him or her. They need to help their child to develop a sense of competency, building on what has gone before, but they should never be afraid to set limits. By getting the little things right, they will ensure that the bigger things are much more likely to be all right, too.

Throughout your child's life, they will learn many things and have many experiences, but the most important of all their influences is you.

Astonishing, isn't it, that we know all of these things already?

Childcare and school: putting change on the agenda

Few would argue that good-quality childcare is essential and can mean the difference between happy, securely attached children and those who are unhappy and anxious. Research tells us that good childcare reduces stress levels in children of working mothers. Sadly, we just don't have enough of this resource to benefit the children who need it.

Once they are at school, children need small classes, which enable everyone to learn, and a flexible curriculum, delivered by teachers who are not bullied into achieving 'standards' and who are not exhausted and demotivated by constantly having to provide data to demonstrate this. Children and teachers benefit from healthy meals during the school day. Children need physical activity – some more than most. Teachers usually know who these children are. Research also suggests that structured environments are better for all children – while they are much needed by some children (usually boys) who are poor at self-regulation, they are not going to disadvantage others.

What stops us achieving these changes? There are not enough teachers and, for the teachers we do have, much of their time is diverted away to non-teaching activities. In affluent countries such as the UK, it should be possible to halve the number of children in each class. We can't do this because public money is being spent on other things. Unfortunately, the government continues to attach a low priority to good universal childcare and schooling experiences, despite a great deal of rhetoric.

We know what conditions are necessary for a healthy body, and we also know a great deal about what is needed for children (and consequently for adults) to be emotionally healthy. We don't need to wait for further 'information', or any kind of 'proof' or new theories or more statistics. We already know what is needed. We also know what isn't – we know that addressing superficial aspects of children's problems (like 'attention') is not helpful while the *real* problems are being ignored. The real problems, we are told, are too difficult and too complex to tackle. Too often, we find ourselves adopting the mantra 'There is no alternative.' *But there is.*

Healthcare choices

The overwhelming majority of children do not need medical responses to their difficulties. There is an urgent need to look at the ways in which children's mental health teams operate and the kind of philosophy that underpins their work. Despite a much increased focus on child and adolescent mental health in recent years and some positive change, in terms of ways of working, it is remarkable how in some ways little has changed. Many children's teams have the same kind of professional 'mix' as they would if they were on a hospital inpatient ward, with psychiatrists, doctors, nurses and occupational therapists making up the core team. These teams are mostly psychiatry led and have a predominantly medical culture. This means that as soon as a child enters the system, he or she is immediately considered through the psychiatric lens. There will be some professional readers of this book who protest at this description of themselves, but I suggest that they are either the exceptions to the rule or that they are so much a part of the system that they have lost the capacity to see it for what it is.

There are some wonderful community teams out there who are pushing the boundaries of innovation and creativity every day. They work in people's homes, in schools, clinics and community centres. They employ counsellors, solution-focused therapists, family workers and other community practitioners who have the skills that match what young people need. They don't need to medicalise them. Unfortunately, because these workers tend to have lower professional status than the traditional 'doctors and nurses' teams, they tend not to be well funded or supported. My experience of the child and adolescent mental health system in the UK is that it does not really encourage psychosocial, non-medical, approaches – you are either subsumed into the medical culture or viewed as a threat (which often means that they will find a way to get rid of you sooner or later). Ironically, psychiatrists are the only professionals who may stray outside these confines and are sometimes allowed to cultivate something of a maverick persona (which generally means that they start to behave like psychologists). This behaviour is usually dismissed as individual eccentricity, which indeed it often is.

Understanding something of the dominant medical culture is important, as this is for the most part a medical story, involving a considerable number of over-enthusiastic psychiatrists. Psychiatry textbooks don't even mention that there is any kind of controversy over ADHD. For newly trained psychiatrists there is only one view, and it has been presented to them with so much certainty that dissension is seen as completely 'off the wall.' I can speak with confidence about this, as I routinely offer training to junior doctors.

Your choice

The NHS is committed to the 'choice' agenda, which means that all of us have a right to the kind of treatment we want for ourselves and for our children (so long as it has a reasonable chance of being effective). As a result, if your child is referred to a child and adolescent mental health service you are entitled to ask about the approach that will be taken with your child, to know who is in the team, and also to know whether they are qualified to do what they say they are doing. If you think that your child has problems with attention, concentration and motivation, you are entitled to ask for a psychological approach (and for a psychologist, if you wish), which might offer a combination of individual work with your child (e.g. cognitive behavioural therapy or solution-focused brief therapy), as well as work with your child's school and possibly also family work, looking at how your family communicates. If you are not offered these things and are offered instead an 'ADHD clinic' or 'medication', you have the right to go somewhere else where you can get more appropriate help.

By now you will have a good idea of my philosophy with regard to children, namely that if we want them to change then we, as the adults, have to be prepared to change first. Genetic and biological explanations offer us nothing of use to help this process of change, either in the sense of our own children and families or in the wider context of the society in which we live.

Jay Joseph, in his book *The Gene Illusion*, uses the disease *pellagra* as an example of an illness which we now know is caused by vitamin deficiency but that was once thought to be genetic. The thing is – and here's the parallel with 'ADHD' – the issue here is not whether or not something is genetic in origin, as we could be waiting 20 more years and still have no definitive 'proof.' But we do know with absolute certainty that we can *all* benefit from a healthy society – just as a healthy diet protects everyone from illness caused by vitamin deficiency.

Joseph reminds his readers of an observation made by biologist Richard Lewontin, who said that the question comes down to whether we see the individual as a problem for society, or society as a problem for the individual. The position adopted by most mental health practitioners who find themselves opposed to 'ADHD' is the result of the evidence that they see before them day in, day out. That evidence tells them that, in an expression much loved by my good friend and colleague, Scott Sinclair, 'the fish ain't sick, the water's dirty.'

A bit of common sense

You will already know, if your child is going through any kind of difficulty or difficult life stage, that at such times you have to keep your parenting 'tight.' Parenting is hard at any time. When there are problems, it's then that you have to rise to the challenge and get even better at it!

The following list contains some common-sense ideas for good parenting that you may or may not already use. They are particularly good for energetic, impulsive children who would rather be doing something else than organise themselves and study.

- A good diet. Try to feed your child good, healthy, fresh food, rather than packaged 'convenience' foods. Fruit and vegetables are essential (five portions a day are recommended). All children need three good meals a day and three healthy snacks. Cut out junk food (sweets, biscuits, chocolates, crisps) and fizzy drinks. Some parents swear by additive-free diets, like the Feingold diet.
- Insist on breakfast for your family (this includes you!). Breakfast together. If you or your child can't face breakfast just after you've woken up, then get up half an hour earlier. Breakfast should be whatever you want it to be, but try to keep it healthy.
- Many parents have found that their children seem to be calmer if they take a fish oil supplement, and research studies have recently supported this view.
- Make sure that your child isn't getting 'hidden' caffeine and stimulants through sports drinks and other 'high-energy' foods.
- Try to ensure that your child has a good sleep routine. A 'set' bedtime is important for all children (see my earlier comments). You can ease up at weekends and allow a later bedtime then.
- Make sure that your child is getting enough exercise and relaxation time, preferably in the fresh air.
- Help your child to organise him- or herself. It doesn't happen by accident and it will be a skill they have for life. You can make a school-days planner together, have it laminated and put it up behind the bedroom door, with a copy downstairs. This

can be checked off every day when bags are packed, etc. Similarly, make sure that you check and sign their homework diary. If your child can get into the habit of forward-planning and doing these things every evening, so that they are ready for the next day, so much the better.

■ This applies to games kit, shoe cleaning, etc. If you do these things for your children, don't be surprised when they don't learn to do them for themselves!

■ Even the youngest children can be helped to sort out their own packed lunch for school.

■ Give your child help with homework, but only ever give *just enough*. The aim is to help your child to become more and more self-sufficient as they get older (not to do the homework yourself so that they/you get high marks). Buy highlighter pens and show them how to use them to pick out important information and instructions. Help them to be clear about what the instructions are asking them to do and how they might answer. To start with, have them near you (the kitchen table is great for little ones). Leave them to it, but keep checking on them to see how they're doing. Extend this with older children, just getting them 'set up' with what they need in their own room (drinks and snacks are much appreciated).

■ Provide positive feedback straight away when you are pleased with something your child has done. Always give praise for good behaviour.

■ Let your child know that you value them. If they make something for you, display it. If they paint you a picture, put it up. Frame your favourites and put them on the wall.

■ Be as good a role model yourself as you can. Try to be calm. Try to be organised.

■ Enjoy your child. Let your enjoyment show. When you do something together and you've enjoyed it, tell them so.

■ All of these things need *time*, so make sure that you've got it.

■ Encourage self-discipline and self-control. Some sports (martial arts and Tai Chi) focus particularly on these skills, but you will need to find a good club.

■ Allow your children to be bored! A lot of parents nowadays rush their children from one activity to another. This is not always good for children, who, just like us, need time to simply relax and do nothing at the end of a long day. I've noticed that parents seem to be particularly keen to 'protect' their children from boredom, so they fill every waking hour for them. This is not necessary. Your child will benefit from learning to amuse him- or herself. When my 12-year-old son broke his leg and had to have some time off school, he took up cooking, walked to the local library using his crutches, took out a book, taught himself html programming and developed his own website for his recipes. Let them discover their own creativity – give them some ideas and support and let them go for it.

■ Look after yourself. If you are part of a couple, make time for your relationship.

What can you do?

If you have enjoyed this book and want to do something about the current ADHD situation, here are some ideas.

1 Write to your MP. If you are not sure who your MP is, you can find out by ringing the House of Commons Public Information Office on 020 7219 4272. You can write to all members of the UK Parliament at: [name] MP, House of Commons, London, SW1A 0AA. Or for members of the Scottish Parliament: [name] MSP, Scottish Parliament, Edinburgh, EH99 1SP.

2 Visit the website for Stimulants Are Not The Answer (SANTA) at: www.santa.inuk.com/action.htm

3 If you are a psychiatrist, get to know the Critical Psychiatry Network, a UK-based network of practising Consultant Psychiatrists who are critical of orthodox beliefs in psychiatry, including those that suggest mental ill-health is caused by underlying brain dysfunctions. They have expressed great concern at the influence of the pharmaceutical companies on mental health perceptions and practice. The Critical Psychiatry Network can be accessed at: www.critpsynet.freeuk.com/

4 Healthy Skepticism is an international organisation for health professionals with an interest in improving health and reducing drug promotion. Visit Health Skepticism at: www.healthyskepticism.org

5 NICE is in the process of developing a clinical guideline on ADHD and is collecting information on 'good practice'. Contact your local Child and Adolescent Mental Health Service and ask to become involved. Your GP practice will have the telephone number.

6 Respond to letters and articles in newspapers and magazines.

7 Let your GP know your views – in writing, if necessary.

8 If your children have grown up and you have any spare capacity to help others, think about becoming a volunteer for an organisation like Home Start, where you could help young parents to cope with parenting.

9 When you vote, make sure that you know each candidate's view on the ADHD issue. Ask them all individually.

10 Make your views known at your child's school or college.

11 Become a school governor.

12 Get involved. There *is* an alternative.

Peter Breggin's critique of the MTA study

Peter Breggin is a well-known psychiatrist in the USA who is sceptical about ADHD as a diagnostic category, and an outspoken critic of drug treatment. Breggin has published a critique of the original National Institute for Mental Health (NIMH) multi-modal treatment study for ADHD (the MTA study), the results of which were published in December 1999.[1,2] This research was widely cited and was very influential in the world of would-be prescribers of stimulant medication for children. Breggin points out that the study had 'several gross methodological flaws that undermine its scientific validity and limit any conclusions that can be drawn from it.'

He lists the following 'flaws.'

1 *The MTA study did not use a placebo (a 'dummy' drug) group, nor did it use a 'double-blind' clinical trial.* Both of these are usually used in studies designed to evaluate the effectiveness of medication, and are accepted methods.

    (The MTA did use one group of 'blinded ratings' in school. The 'blind' raters found no difference between any of the treatment groups on any of the variables involving ADHD or oppositional behaviour. However, this finding was excluded from the conclusions of the study.)

2 *The study had no 'control group' of untreated children.* Again, research studies such as this one, looking at the effectiveness of a drug, would usually be expected to have one. Children who had been treated with medication could not therefore be compared with children who had not.

3 *The researchers relied on parent and teacher evaluations.*

4 *32% of the medication management group was already on medication for ADHD at the start of the MTA.*

    As Breggin notes, this is 'generally not acceptable in a study of medication effects and would be expected to corrupt the study.' He adds, 'since the children were already receiving medication, it is highly probable that their parents had already determined to their own satisfaction that the drugs were helpful. Therefore they could not participate objectively in a "random" drug study.'

5 *The medication management group was highly selective.* Children were recruited from a wide range of sources, such as clinics, schools and public advertisements.

However, of 4,541 children, only 579 (12.8%) were selected for the trials. As already noted, many of these were already taking stimulant medication.

6 *The medication management group was relatively small.* Only 144 of the 579 children accepted; 13 of these dropped out before starting, and a further eight dropped out during the study. 'Overall, of the 4,541 children originally screened, only 12.8% entered the study and only 2.7% (123 children) completed the medication management trial.

7 *Children did not rate themselves as improved.* The children rated themselves on anxiety (no change). In addition, however, Breggin claims to have received information that the children also rated themselves on depression and that this was confirmed by a handout provided by the New York State Psychiatric Institute and Columbia University Division of Child and Adolescent Psychiatry in 1994. However, the MTA reports no data on the children's depression ratings. As Breggin points out, this is an important omission, as stimulants commonly cause depression in children. He asks, 'Were the depression self-rating scales dropped because they indicated a worsening of the children's condition?'

8 *Most of the children in the MTA (80%) were boys.* Breggin points out that stimulants are known to be temporarily effective in suppressing spontaneous behaviour in children and animals, and suggests that it is this suppression of socialisation, play, autonomy and spontaneity that makes 'normal' boys easier to manage in classroom or home environments that do not meet their needs for spontaneous activity, fail to engage them in education or do not provide consistent discipline within the family setting.

9 *The behavioural treatments were flawed.* The behavioural treatments were developed by Russell Barkley and have been criticised as being 'limited.'

10 *Most children suffered adverse drug reactions (ADRs).* In total, 64% of children were reported to have ADRs (11.4% 'moderate' and 2.9% 'severe').

11 *There were no trained observers for ADRs.* Breggin adds, 'Furthermore, many ADRs – such as behavioural suppression, loss of spontaneity, apathy and increased obsessive behaviour – are mistakenly interpreted as improvements by parents and teachers.'

12 *There was no improvement in academic performance.*

13 *There was very little effect on social skills.*

14 *All of the principal investigators were well-known drug advocates.*

15 *The parents and teachers were exposed to pro-drug propaganda.*

Comparison of 1997 Labour Party Manifesto with position and plans in 2006

This table is adapted from an original produced by Sheila Porter-Williams for the Campaign for Health Service Democracy. She is contactable at: Sheila@healthdemocracy.org.uk. It is accessible at: www.healthdemocracy.org.uk/.../Comparison%202006%20against%201997%20Labour%20Party%20Manifesto.htm

The table compares extracts on the NHS from the 1997 Labour Party Manifesto with the position and plans in 2006. Many of the policies have failed or been reversed.

1997 Labour Party Manifesto	Position and plans in 2006
In health policy, we will safeguard the basic principles of the NHS, which we founded, but will not return to the top-down management of the 1970s. So we will keep the planning and provision of healthcare separate, but put planning on a longer-term, decentralised and more co-operative basis. The key is to root out unnecessary administrative costs, and to spend money on the right things – frontline care. Over the five years of a Labour government: We will rebuild the NHS, reducing spending on administration and increasing spending on patient care. We will save the NHS.	**Policy failed.** Administrative costs have increased. Management structures are reorganised every few years, so each local body achieves very little apart from implementing centrally determined policies. Local accountability of NHS bodies is limited, and there is no local democratic decision making on decisions like closures of community hospitals. Complex financial interrelationships and centrally imposed contracts and policies have led to some (possibly a majority) of local NHS bodies being unable to sustain their current level of front-line services within their budgets, even though resources allocated have increased substantially.
100,000 people off waiting lists.	Reductions in waiting lists were achieved. In part this was through creation of surplus capacity in the extremely expensive Independent-Sector Treatment Centres, some of whose surgeons have botched operations that have had to be redone or have left patients damaged. In part the reduction in waiting lists was achieved by manipulation of figures by staff in NHS trusts, with passive acceptance at strategic health authority level.

1997 Labour Party Manifesto	Position and plans in 2006
End the Tory internal market.	**Policy reversed.** The internal market has evolved, but is still an expensive bureaucracy distorting decisions at all levels.
End waiting for cancer surgery.	Achieved, although there is a risk that progress will be lost as a result of service cuts affecting most of the country, due to misdirected resources.
Tough quality targets for hospitals.	Waiting-time targets have in part distorted priorities away from seriously ill patients and resulted in scarcity of emergency beds and long ambulance journeys for critically injured patients. See routine service failures.
Independent food standards agency.	The Food Standards Agency was established, although it has had to resist political pressure to suppress bad news.
New public health drive.	Dangerous when it has led to denial of treatment for people with supposedly unhealthy lifestyles.
Raise spending in real terms every year – and spend the money on patients, not bureaucracy.	Spending has increased, and patients have benefited to some extent. Some of the extra spending has been on surplus capacity, expensive contracts and increased bureaucracy, while mainstream services have been cut because of incompetent budgeting at national level.
Labour created the NHS 50 years ago. It is under threat from the Conservatives. We want to save and modernise the NHS. But if the Conservatives are elected again there may well not be an NHS in five years' time – either national or comprehensive. Labour commits itself anew to the historic principle that if you are ill or injured there will be a national health service there to help, and access to it will be based on need and need alone – not on your ability to pay, or on who your GP happens to be, or on where you live.	There are contradictions in government policy. The Choose and Book policy will when fully developed mean that patients will be able to go to any hospital in the country, at least for elective surgery. The National Institute for Health and Clinical Excellence is established to advise on which treatments should be used, but its research capacity was cut in 2005, causing a backlog, and some of its recommendations appear to be influenced more by the cost of a treatment than by its efficacy. Policies of primary care trusts differ, and some limit access to treatments on arbitrary grounds (such as unhealthy lifestyles) or deny access to expensive new potentially life-saving treatments while they prioritise cutting waiting times for elective surgery for conditions that are inconvenient and/or painful but not life-threatening. Postcode prescribing is still thriving.

1997 Labour Party Manifesto	Position and plans in 2006
In 1990 the Conservatives imposed on the NHS a complex internal market of hospitals competing to win contracts from health authorities and fundholding GPs. The result is an NHS strangled by costly red tape, with every individual transaction the subject of a separate invoice. After six years, bureaucracy swallows an extra £1.5 billion per year, there are 20,000 more managers and 50,000 fewer nurses on the wards, and more than one million people are on waiting lists. The government has consistently failed to meet even its own health targets. There can be no return to top-down management, but Labour will end the Conservatives' internal market in healthcare. The planning and provision of care are necessary and distinct functions, and will remain so. But under the Tories, the administrative costs of purchasing care have undermined provision and the market system has distorted clinical priorities. Labour will cut costs by removing the bureaucratic processes of the internal market.	The separation of commissioning and provision for acute and community services is costly, and diverts resources from patient care. **Policy reversed.** The latest phase of the internal market is payment by results, with money following the patients. The system is destabilising (liable to randomly shift deficits between acute trusts and primary care trusts, so that nobody knows the consolidated deficit and services to patients will be unnecessarily cut), open to manipulation and costly to administer. The tariff for payment by results is substantially exceeded by contractual payments for Independent Sector Treatment Centres, and unable to support the costs of hospitals funded through the Private Finance Initiative.
The savings achieved will go on direct care for patients. As a start, the first £100 million saved will treat an extra 100,000 patients.	**Policy failed.** No significant savings were achieved. Extra resources have been allocated. Much of the benefit has been lost by badly costed changes in contracts for NHS workers, creation of expensive surplus capacity in the private sector to reduce waiting times for elective surgery, and unnecessary changes in the management structures that can only have increased costs. The effect on costs of new, more effective but much more expensive treatments has been underestimated.
We will end waiting for cancer surgery, thereby helping thousands of women waiting for breast cancer treatment.	Achieved, although there is a risk that progress will be lost as a result of service cuts affecting most of the country due to misdirected resources.
Primary care will play a lead role. In recent years, GPs have gained power on behalf of their patients in a changed relationship with consultants, and we support this. But the development of GP fundholding has also brought disadvantages. Decision making has been fragmented. Administrative costs have grown. And a two-tier service has resulted.	**Policy failed.** The primary care groups foreshadowed here were short-lived and were replaced by larger primary care trusts, which in 2006 are due to be merged to boundaries similar to the pre-1997 health authorities – an expensive diversion of effort away from direct patient care. It is dangerous to give any professional group too much power in the administration of the NHS.

1997 Labour Party Manifesto	Position and plans in 2006
Labour will retain the lead role for primary care but remove the disadvantages that have come from the present system. GPs and nurses will take the lead in combining together locally to plan local health services more efficiently for all the patients in their area.	See Sharon Wilson for where a primary care trust has colluded in the black-listing of a seriously ill patient whose complaints against various GPs have not been mutually resolved.
This will enable all GPs in an area to bring their combined strength to bear upon individual hospitals to secure higher standards of patient provision. In making this change, we will build on the existing collaborative schemes which already serve 14 million people. The current system of year-on-year contracts is costly and unstable. We will introduce three- to five-year agreements between the local primary care teams and hospitals. Hospitals will then be better able to plan work at full capacity and co-operate to enhance patient services.	**Policy reversed.** The Choose and Book system will give patients choice as to which hospitals or private clinics they use for elective surgery, so there will be no contractual commitment to send elective surgery patients to the local hospital, and the finances of hospital trusts will be destabilised. At least patients will be able to choose the local hospital, where previous contracts may have been less convenient for people living in some areas. In the Choose and Book system, local commissioning adds cost, complexity and inconsistent policies (postcode prescribing) to no benefit.
Higher-quality services for patients. Hospitals will retain their autonomy over day-to-day administrative functions, but, as part of the NHS, they will be required to meet high-quality standards in the provision of care. Management will be held to account for performance levels.	The original star ratings ignored hospitals' relative quality of outcome, and concentrated on secondary but more easily measured issues such as waiting times. The ratings were unstable, and a hospital or other trust could move up or down the ratings by two stars in a single year, although it is unlikely that any hospital would improve or deteriorate so fast. The new 2005 system of self-assessment at least has the advantage of encouraging hospitals to identify and correct their own weaknesses rather than dispute a rating by an outside body.
Boards will become more representative of the local communities that they serve.	**Policy failed.** No progress except in foundation trusts, which are inappropriate bodies for direct election because relatively few people have a long-term relationship with an acute hospital. It is the primary care trusts that should be directly elected and should control the acute hospitals, etc.
A new patients' charter will concentrate on the quality and success of treatment.	The Government has not produced a new patients' charter. The Campaign for Health Service Democracy has prepared a statement of citizen's rights in the NHS.
The Tories' so-called 'Efficiency Index' counts the number of patient 'episodes', not the quality or success of treatment. With Labour, the measure will be quality of outcome, itself an incentive for effectiveness.	It is difficult to measure quality of outcome because the figures need to be weighted according to how ill patients were in the first instance. There have been few official figures, but some weighted performance figures have been published, mainly in the press. See clinical outcomes.

1997 Labour Party Manifesto	Position and plans in 2006
As part of our concern to ensure quality, we will work towards the elimination of mixed-sex wards.	As old large wards are closed and replaced by wards consisting of smaller bays or single rooms, this will be a natural consequence.
Health authorities will become the guardians of high standards. They will monitor services, spread best practice and ensure rising standards of care.	This role has gone to new bodies such as the Healthcare Commission. Commissioning primary care trusts have accountability for standards with minimal influence to improve them.
The Tory attempt to use private money to build hospitals has failed to deliver. Labour will overcome the problems that have plagued the Private Finance Initiative, end the delays, sort out the confusion and develop new forms of public/private partnership that work better and protect the interests of the NHS.	**Policy failed.** Running costs of new hospitals financed through the Private Finance Initiative are unaffordable unless specially subsidised, and some schemes have been delayed or curtailed at a late stage for reasons of unaffordability. The Local Improvement Finance Trust (LIFT) does not have the same problem because it is used for primary care, which is not under the same financial pressure.
Labour is opposed to the privatisation of clinical services which is being actively promoted by the Conservatives.	**Policy reversed.** Elective surgery has been contracted to multinational companies through Independent-Sector Treatment Centres, which are expensive and sometimes incompetent, and have surplus capacity whose cost has diverted resources from treatments that are more clinically urgent. Some primary care has been contracted to multinational companies instead of the traditional local professional practices.
Labour will promote new developments in telemedicine – bringing expert advice from regional centres of excellence to neighbourhood level using new technology.	NHS Direct is a quiet success, although under-resourced and insufficiently publicised. Patients who actually need to see a doctor out of hours have a great variety of arrangements across the country, often involving numerous telephone calls.
Good health. A new minister for public health will attack the root causes of ill health, and so improve lives and save the NHS money. Labour will set new goals for improving the overall health of the nation which recognise the impact that poverty, poor housing, unemployment and a polluted environment have on health.	Partial success. Unhealthy lifestyles have not changed greatly, and improvement has been hampered by long-term contracts to sell junk food at schools. The impetus to change this came not from politicians, but from a celebrity chef. A pernicious move has been the threat, and sometimes reality, of denial of NHS treatment to people with conditions that may have been caused by unhealthy lifestyles.

1997 Labour Party Manifesto	Position and plans in 2006
Smoking is the greatest single cause of preventable illness and premature death in the UK. We will therefore ban tobacco advertising.	**Policy compromised and delayed.** Tobacco sponsorship of Formula One motor racing was permitted for several years after lobbying by a former Labour Party donor. This temporary exemption was extended to snooker. Subsequently, and after a faltering start, legislation was brought forward to ban smoking in enclosed public spaces.
Labour will establish an independent food standards agency. The £3.5 billion BSE crisis and the *E.coli* outbreak, which resulted in serious loss of life, have made unanswerable the case for the independent agency we have proposed.	The Food Standards Agency was established, although it has had to resist political pressure to suppress bad news regarding the possible pollution of milk when animal carcasses were being cremated out of doors during the recent outbreak of foot and mouth disease. Progress in improving food labelling has been slow.
NHS spending. The Conservatives have wasted spending on the NHS. We will do better. We will raise spending on the NHS in real terms every year and put the money towards patient care. And a greater proportion of every pound spent will go on patient care, not bureaucracy.	**Policy failed.** Extra resources have been allocated, but much of the benefit has been lost by badly costed changes in contracts for NHS workers, creation of expensive surplus capacity in the private sector to reduce waiting times for elective surgery, and unnecessary changes in the management structures that can only have increased costs. The effect on costs of new, more effective but much more expensive treatments has been underestimated.
An NHS for the future. The NHS requires continuity as well as change, or the system cannot cope. There must be pilots to ensure that change works. And there must be flexibility, not rigid prescription, if innovation is to flourish. Our fundamental purpose is simple but hugely important: to restore the NHS as a public service working co-operatively for patients, not a commercial business driven by competition.	**Policy reversed.** Untried policies that have been hastily imposed throughout England include: Independent Sector Treatment Centres; Choose and Book, with money following the patient according to an untested tariff, and unpredictable consequences in service cuts in some areas; primary care trusts replacing larger district health authorities; local medical and dental practices losing responsibility for out-of-hours care, with no evaluation of the cost to primary care trusts of making provision; primary care trusts merged, often to previous district health authority boundaries.

References

Chapter 1

1 Taylor E, Sandberg S, Thorley G *et al*. *The Epidemiology of Childhood Hyperactivity*. Maudsley Monograph. London: Oxford University Press; 1991.

2 Rowland AS, Lesesne CA, Abramowitz AJ. The epidemiology of attention deficit/hyperactivity disorder (ADHD): a public health view. *Ment Retard Dev Disabil Res Rev*. 2002; 8: 162–70.

3 McArdle P, O'Brien G, Kolvin I. Hyperactivity: prevalence and relationship with conduct disorder. *J Child Psychol Psychiatry*. 1995; 36: 279–303.

4 Gaub M, Carlson CL. Gender differences in ADHD: a meta-analysis and critical review. *J Am Acad Child Adolesc Psychiatry*. 1997; 36: 1036.

5 Blashfield RK. Predicting DSM-V. *J Nerv Ment Dis*. 1996; 184: 4–7.

6 Lenzer J. Untitled update on MindFreedom International News, 24 October 2005; www.oikos.org/antipsychiatry/2004dendrite34.htm (accessed 8 August 2006).

7 Timimi S. *Pathological Child Psychiatry and the Medicalization of Childhood*. Hove: Brunner-Routledge; 2002.

8 Breggin P. *Toxic Psychiatry*. London: Harper Collins; 1993.

9 Bentall R. *Madness Explained: psychosis and human nature in medicine*. Harmondsworth: Penguin; 2003.

10 Bentall R, op. cit.

11 Mental Health Foundation. The information in this fact sheet is taken from a variety of sources, including *Fundamental Facts: All the Latest Facts and Figures on Mental Illness*, published by the Mental Health Foundation in 1999. It was last updated on 2 July 2003. Available at www.mental health.org.uk (accessed 20 April 2006).

12 Joseph J. *The Gene Illusion: genetic research in psychiatry and psychology under the microscope*. New York: Algora Publishing; 2004.

13 Joseph J, op. cit.

14 Lewis T, Amini F, Lannon R. *A General Theory of Love*. New York: Random House; 2000.

15 Sherman DK, Iacono WG, McGue MK. Attention-deficit hyperactivity disorder dimensions: a twin study of inattention and impulsivity–hyperactivity. *J Am Acad Child Adolesc Psychiatry*. 1997; 36: 745–53; Edelbrock C *et al*. A twin study of competence and problem behavior in childhood and early adolescence. *J Child Psychol Psychiatry*. 1995; 36: 775–86.

16 Joseph J, op. cit.
17 Galves A, Walker DD. *Debunking the Science Behind ADHD as a 'Brain Disorder.'* Washington, DC: Academy for the Study of the Psychoanalytic Arts, American Psychological Association; 2002.
18 Thomas A, Chess S. *Temperament and Development.* New York: Brunner-Mazel; 1977.
19 Barkley R, Cook EH, Dulcan M *et al.* International Consensus Statement on ADHD; www.addwarehouse.com (accessed 20 April 2006).
20 Moncrieff J. *Is Psychiatry for Sale?* London: Institute of Psychiatry; 2003.
21 Timimi S. *Naughty Boys.* Basingstoke: Palgrave Macmillan; 2005.

Chapter 2

1 Gaub M, Carlson CL. Gender differences in ADHD: a meta-analysis and critical review. *J Am Acad Child Adolesc Psychiatry.* 1997; **36**: 1036.
2 Nikkhah R. Alarm as prescriptions of Ritalin reach a record high. *The Daily Telegraph,* 20 September 2005.
3 All of these figures have been provided by the House of Commons written answers for July 2003. Available at www.publications.parliament.uk (accessed 20 April 2006).
4 Nikkah R, op. cit.
5 Burne J. Mother's Little Helper. *The Guardian,* 3 March 2005.
6 Nikkhah R, op. cit.
7 International Narcotics Control Board. *Annual Report. Press Release No. 4,* 23 February 2000.
8 Green H, McGinnity A, Meltzer H *et al. Mental Health of Children and Young People in Great Britain, 2004.* Basingstoke: Palgrave Macmillan; 2005.
9 Anon. Ritalin rise leads to ADHD probe. BBC Scotland news item, 20 December 2004; http://news.bbc.co.uk/1/hi/scotland (accessed 7 July 2006).
10 Berbatis CG, Sunderland VB, Bulsara M. Licit psychostimulant consumption in Australia, 1984–2000: international and jurisdictional comparison. *Med J Aust.* 2002; **177**: 539–43.
11 Volkow ND, Ding U, Fowler JS *et al.* Is methylphenidate like cocaine? Studies on their pharmacokinetics and distribution in the human brain. *Arch Gen Psychiatry.* 1995; **52**: 456–62.
12 Volkow ND, Wang GJ, Fowler JS *et al.* Therapeutic doses of oral methylphenidate significantly increase extracellular dopamine in the human brain. *J Neurosci.* 2001; **21**: 1–5.
13 Jackson GE. Food and Drug Administration Hearings on Stimulants, 23 March 2006. Available at: http://icspp.org/pdf/JacksonMDcommentaryfor23march2006.pdf
14 Cross CR. *Heavier Than Heaven: the biography of Kurt Cobain.* London: Hodder and Stoughton; 2001.
15 Wurtzel E. *More, Now, Again.* London: Virago; 2003.
16 Jackson G. *Rethinking Psychiatric Drugs: a guide for informed consent.* Bloomington, IN: AuthorHouse; 2005.
17 Baughman F. *History of the Fraud of Biological Psychiatry;* www.adhdfraud.org/history_of_the_fraud_of_biological_psychiatry.htm (accessed 8 August 2006).
18 Gordons E. *The American Children's Silent Deaths;* www.thepetitionsite.com (accessed 8 August 2006).
19 Zito JM, Safer DJ, dosReis S *et al.* Trends in the prescribing of psychotropic medications to preschoolers. *JAMA.* 2000; **283**: 1025–30.
20 Nikkah R, op. cit.

21 Vidal G. *Perpetual War for Perpetual Peace: how we got to be so hated.* Forest Row, East Sussex: Clairview Books, Temple Lodge Publishing; 2002.

22 Jackson G. *What doctors may not tell you about psychiatric drugs.* Transcript from Public Lecture, Centre for Community Mental Health, University of Central England in Birmingham, 9 June 2004.

23 Breggin P. *Toxic Psychiatry. Drugs and electroconvulsive therapy: the truth and the better alternatives.* London: Harper Collins; 1993.

24 McDonagh MS, Peterson K. *Drug Class Review on Pharmacologic Treatments for ADHD.* Portland, OR: Oregon Evidence-based Practice Center, Oregon Health and Science University, 2006; www.ohsu.edu/drugeffectiveness/reports/final.cfm

Chapter 3

1 Harris G. As doctors write prescriptions, drug company writes a check. *New York Times*, 27 June 2004.

2 Spence D. *The Influence of the Pharmaceutical Industry.* House of Commons Health Committee. Formal minutes, oral and written evidence. London: The Stationery Office; 2005.

3 Katz D, Caplan AL, Merz JF. All gifts large and small: towards an understanding of the ethics of pharmaceutical industry gift-giving. *Am J Bioethics.* 2003; 3: 39–46.

4 Shaughnessy AF, Slawson DC. Pharmaceutical representatives. *BMJ.* 1996; 312: 1494.

5 Boseley S. Drug firm censured for lapdancing junket. *The Guardian*, 14 February 2006.

6 Spence D, op. cit.

7 Dowd J. *The Influence of the Pharmaceutical Industry.* House of Commons Health Committee. Formal minutes, oral and written evidence. London: The Stationery Office; 2005.

8 BBC Radio 4. *You and Yours*, 22 November 2004; www.bbc.co.uk/radio4/youandyours/index_20041122.shtml

9 Deutsche Bank Mid-Cap Life Sciences, Services and Devices Conference, 27 June 2003. Shire Pharmaceuticals group plc; www.shire.com/shire/uploads/presentations/DB_Conf_270603.pdf (accessed 1 March 2007).

10 O'Meara KP. Doping Kids. *Insight on the News*, 28 June 1999.

11 Spence D, op. cit.

12 Harris G, op. cit.

13 Ross JS, Lurie P, Wolfe SM. Health Research Group Report: medical education services suppliers – a threat to physician education. *Public Citizen*, 19 July 2000; www.citizen.org/publications/release.cfm (accessed 14 September 2006).

14 Templeton SK. Drug firm bias causes wrong diagnosis. *The Sunday Herald*, 16 June 2006; www.sundayherald.com/25489 (accessed 14 September 2006).

15 Harding A. European and US groups draw up standards for CME. *BMJ.* 2004; 328: 1279.

16 Bodenheimer T. Uneasy alliance – clinical investigations and the pharmaceutical industry. *NEJM.* 2000; 342: 1539.

17 Angell M. Is academic medicine for sale? *NEJM.* 2000; 342: 1516–18.

18 Moncrieff J. *Is Psychiatry for Sale?* Maudsley Discussion Paper. London: Institute of Psychiatry; 2003.

19 Wilmshurst P. *The Influence of the Pharmaceutical Industry.* House of Commons Health Committee. Formal minutes, oral and written evidence. London: The Stationery Office; 2005.

20 Wilmshurst P, ibid.

21 Wilmshurst P, ibid.
22 Wilmshurst P, ibid.
23 Harris G, op. cit.
24 No Free Lunch – UK. *The Influence of the Pharmaceutical Industry.* Submission to the House of Commons Health Committee. Formal minutes, oral and written evidence. London: The Stationery Office; 2005.
25 Hearn K. USA: drug companies pushing ADHD drugs for children. CorpWatch, November 2004; www.corpwatch.org (accessed 14 July 2006).
26 Osman K, Parker J. ADHD: how are specialist nurses doing? *Child Adolesc Ment Health Prim Care.* 2003; 1: 82–4.
27 Osman K, Parker J, ibid.
28 Celltech Pharmaceuticals Inc. *A Teacher's Guide to ADHD and Methylphenidate.* Rochester, NY: Celltech Pharmaceuticals Inc; 2004.
29 National Attention Deficit Disorder Information and Support Service (ADDISS). *ADHD: paying enough attention. A research report investigating ADHD in the UK;* www.addiss.co.uk/factsheets.htm (accessed 14 July 2006).
30 Shamim W, Yousufuddin M, Wang D *et al.* Nonsurgical reduction of the interventricular septum in patients with hypertrophic cardiomyopathy *NEJM.* 2002; **347:** 1326–33. Retraction published in *NEJM.* 2003; **348:** 10.
31 Barnett A. Revealed: how drug firms 'hoodwink' medical journals. *The Observer,* 7 December 2003.
32 Doward J, McKie R. Dark secrets lurking in the drugs cabinet. *The Observer,* 7 November 2004.
33 Barnett A, op. cit.
34 Barnett A, op. cit.
35 Barnett A, op. cit.
36 Hearn K. *Here, Kiddie, Kiddie.* AlterNet, November 2004; http://alternet.org/drugreporter/20594/ (accessed 12 July 2006).
37 Hearn K, ibid.
38 Moncrieff J, op. cit.
39 White M. On May 1 Paul Drayson was given a peerage. On June 17 he gave Labour a £500,000 cheque. *The Guardian,* 25 August 2004.
40 Willman D. US scientists' deal with drug firms under review. *The Los Angeles Times,* 7 December 2003.
41 Moncrieff J, op. cit.

Chapter 4

1 Peart RF. *The Benzodiazepines: transcript of verbal submission to the Select Committee on Health Inquiry.* House of Commons Health Committee Inquiry on Procedures Related to Adverse Clinical Incidents and Outcomes in Medical Care, June 1999; www.benzo.org.uk (accessed 2 August 2006).
2 Gerada C, Ashforth M. ABC of Mental Health. Addiction and dependence: illicit drugs. *BMJ.* 1997; **315:** 287–300.
3 Committee on Safety of Medicines. *Benzodiazepines: dependence and withdrawal symptoms;* www.benzo.org.uk (accessed 2 August 2006).
4 Department of Health. *National Service Framework for Mental Health: modern service standards and service models.* (30 September 1999); www.dh.gov.uk/en/

publicationsandstatistics/publications/publicationspolicyandguidance/DH_4009598 (accessed 22 April 2006).

5 Department of Health. *Benzodiazepines Warning: a communication to all doctors from the Chief Medical Officer's Update 37*; www.benzo.org.uk/cmo.htm (accessed 2 August 2006).

6 Jackson G. *What doctors may not tell you about psychiatric drugs.* Transcript from Public Lecture, Centre for Community Mental Health, University of Central England in Birmingham, 9 June 2004; www.ccmh.uce.ac.uk/dr_%20grace_%20jackson_transcript_09.06.04.pdf (accessed 2 August 2006).

7 Kirsch I, Moore TJ, Scoboria A *et al.* The emperor's new drugs: an analysis of antidepressant medication data submitted to the US Food and Drug Administration. *Prev Treatment.* 2002a; **5**: Article 23.

8 Press Association. *SSRI dangers for children 'suppressed.'* 23 April 2004.

9 Saz EJ, De-las-Cuevas C, Kiuru A *et al.* Selective serotonin reuptake inhibitors in pregnant women and neonatal withdrawal symptoms. *Lancet.* 2005; **365**: 482–7.

10 Wen SW, Yang Q, Garner P *et al.* Selective serotonin reuptake inhibitors and adverse pregnancy outcomes. *Am J Obstet Gynecol.* 2006; **194**: 961–6.

11 Press Association, op. cit.

12 Boseley S. Company 'held back' data on drug for children: anti-depressant had no effect, leak reveals. *The Guardian*, 3 February 2004.

13 Townsend M. Stay calm everyone, there's Prozac in the drinking water. *The Observer*, 8 August 2004.

14 Zito JM, Safer DJ, dos Reis S *et al.* Trends in the prescribing of psychotropic drugs to pre-schoolers. *JAMA.* 2000; **283**: 1025–30.

15 Ornstein R, Sorbel D. *The Healing Brain.* London: Macmillan; 1989.

16 Moncrieff J. *Is Psychiatry for Sale?* Maudsley Discussion Paper. London: Institute of Psychiatry; 2003.

17 Moncrieff J, ibid.

18 Lenzer J. Bush plans to screen whole US population for mental illness. *BMJ.* 2004; **328**: 1458.

19 Lenzer J. Whistleblower charges medical oversight bureau with corruption. *BMJ.* 2004; **329**: 69.

20 Taylor R, Giles J. Cash interests taint drug advice. *Nature.* 2005; **437**: 1070–1.

21 Taylor R, Giles J, ibid.

22 Taylor R, Giles J, ibid.

23 Moncrieff J, op cit.

Chapter 5

1 Rosemund J. *The ADD–TV Connection Affirmed.* Raleigh, NC: The News & Observer; 1997.

2 Kubey R. *Creating Television: conversations with the people behind 50 years of American television.* Mahwah, NJ: Lawrence Erlbaum Associates; 2004.

3 Holt J. *How Children Fail.* Harmondsworth: Pelican Books; 1984.

Chapter 6

1 Green H, McGinnity A, Meltzer H *et al.* *Mental Health of Children and Young People in Great Britain, 2004.* Basingstoke: Palgrave Macmillan; 2005.

2 Flury J. *Ritalin Ripple Effect*; www.educationnews.org (accessed 20 April 2006).

3 Bowlby J. *Attachment and Loss. Volume 1. Attachment.* New York: Basic Books; 1969.

4 Hartmann T. *Attention Deficit Disorder: a different perception (a hunter in a farmer's world)*. Nevada: Underwood Books; 1997.

5 Matajcek Z. Is ADHD adaptive or non-adaptive behaviour? *Neuroendocrinol Lett.* 2003; **24**: 148–50.

6 MacDonald K. Evolution and development. In: Campbell A, Muncer S, editors. *Social Development.* London: UCL Press; 1998. pp. 21–49.

7 Johnston C. Male teachers don't benefit boys, study finds. *Education Guardian*, 9 September 2005.

8 Pollock W. *Real Boys: rescuing our boys from the myths of boyhood.* New York: Henry Holt and Company; 1998.

9 Pollock W, ibid.

10 Timimi S. *Naughty Boys.* Basingstoke: Palgrave Macmillan; 2005.

11 Flury J. *Ritalin Ripple Effect*; www.educationnews.org (accessed 20 April 2006); Whitehorn B. *Raising Boys' Achievement.* Okehampton: Devon Curriculum Services, Okehampton College; 2002; www.devon.gov.uk.des/a/boys/info.doc (accessed 16 June 2006); Hutton W. Boys today? We're doing their heads in. *The Observer*, 4 June 2006.

12 Whitehorn B. *Raising Boys' Achievement.* Okehampton: Devon Curriculum Services, Okehampton College; 2002; www.devon.gov.uk.des/a/boys/info.doc (accessed 16 June 2006).

13 Flury J. *Ritalin Ripple Effect*; www.educationnews.org (accessed 20 April 2006).

14 Flury J, ibid.

15 Timimi S, op. cit.

16 Green H, McGinnity A, Meltzer H *et al.*, op. cit.

17 Katyal S, Awasthi E. Gender differences in emotional intelligence among adolescents of Chandigarh. *J Hum Ecology.* 2005; **17**: 153–5.

18 Charbonneau D, Nicol AA. Emotional intelligence and pro-social behaviours in adolescents. *Psychol Rep.* 2002; **90**: 361–70.

19 Kindlon D, Thompson M. *Raising Cain.* New York: Ballantine Books; 2000.

20 Hutton W. Boys today? We're doing their heads in. *The Observer*, 4 June 2006.

21 Pyke N. How should we teach boys? *The Independent*, 12 September 2002.

22 Pyke N, ibid.

23 Whitehorn B, op. cit.

24 Pyke N, op. cit.

25 Wendt M. *Kids Running. How running and exercise can impact on behaviour of ADHD children*; http://kidsrunning.com/krnews0131adhd.html (accessed 2 August 2006).

26 Department of Education and Science. *Raising Boys' Achievement*; www.dfes.gov.uk/research/data/uploadfiles/RR636.pdf (accessed 2 August 2006).

27 Wiseman B. Testimony presented to the Pennsylvania House Democratic Policy Committee, Philadelphia, Pennsylvania, 20 July 1999; www.thetruthseeker.co.uk/print.asp?ID=27 (accessed 2 August 2006).

28 Economic and Social Research Council. *Facts and Figures. UK Factsheet: violence in the UK*; www.esrcsocietytoday.ac.uk?ESRCInfoCentre/facts/UK/index28.aspx?ComponentID=7103&.SourcePageId=14975 (accessed 2 August 2006).

29 Economic and Social Research Council. *Facts and Figures. UK Factsheet: crime in the UK*; www.esrcsocietytoday.ac.uk?ESRCInfoCentre/facts/UK/index28.aspx?ComponentID=7037&SourcePageID=14975 (accessed 2 August 2006).

30 US Department of Justice. *Office of Justice Program. Homicide trends in the US, June 2006*; www.ojp.usdoj.gov/bjs/homicide/homtmd.htm (accessed 22 July 2006).

31 *Zero Tolerance Policy Report. Final Report of Bi-Partisan Working Group on Youth Violence*, 106th Congress, February 2000.

32 Green H, McGinnity A, Meltzer H *et al.*, op. cit.

Chapter 7

1 Winnicott DW. *Through Pediatrics to Psychoanalysis*. New York: Basic Books; 1952.

2 National Institute for Clinical Excellence. *Guidance on the Use of Methylphenidate (Ritalin, Equasym) for Attention Deficit Hyperactivity Disorder (ADHD)*; www.nice.org. uk/page.aspx?o=11652 (accessed 22 July 2006).

3 Lupien SJ, King S, Meaney MJ *et al.* Can poverty get under your skin? Basal cortisol levels and cognitive function in children from low and high socio-economic status. *Dev Psychopathol*. 2001; **13**: 653–76.

4 Lupien SJ, Fiocco A, Wan N *et al.* Stress hormones and human memory function across the lifespan. *Psychoneuroendocrinology*. 2006; **31**: 142–3.

5 Nachmias M, Gunnar M, Mangelsdorf S *et al.* Behavioural inhibition and stress reactivity: the moderating role of attachment security. *Child Dev*. 1996; **67**: 508–22.

6 Gunnar MR. Stress reactivity and attachment security. *Dev Psychobiol*. 1996; **29**: 191–204. Gunnar MR. Quality of care and buffering of neuroendocrine stress reactions: potential effects on the developing brain. *Prev Med*. 1998; **27**: 208–11.

7 Deutsch CK, Swanson JM, Bruell JH *et al.* Over-representation of adoptees in children with attention deficit disorder. *Behav Genet*. 1982; **12**: 231–8.

8 O'Connor TG, Schlomo YB, Heron J *et al.* Prenatal anxiety predicts individual differences in cortisol in pre-adolescent children. *Biol Psychiatry*. 2005; **58**: 211–17.

9 Selemon LD, Wang L, Nebel MB *et al.* Direct and indirect effects of fetal irradiation on cortical gray and white matter volume in the Macaque. *Biol Psychiatry*, 2005; **57**: 83–90.

10 Torrey FE, Rawlings R, Yoken RH. The antecedents of psychoses: a case–control study of selected risk factors. *Schizophr Res*. 2000; **30**: 17–23.

11 Balista AM, McCreadie RG, Cimmino C *et al.* Can breastfeeding protect against schizophrenia? *Biol Neonate*. 2003; **83**: 97–101.

Chapter 8

1 Hoshi Y, Onoe H, Watanabe Y *et al.* Non-synchronous behaviour of neuronal activity, oxidative metabolism and blood supply during mental tasks in man. *Neurosci Lett*. 1994; **172**: 129–33.

2 Phillips H. 'Rewired brain' revives patient after 19 years. *New Scientist*, 3 July 2006.

3 Gopnick A, Meltzoff A, Kuhl P. *The Scientist in the Crib: what early learning tells us about the mind*. New York: Harper Collins; 1999.

4 Greenough WT, Black JE. Induction of brain structure by experience: substrates for cognitive development. In: Gunnar MR, Nelson CA, editors. *Minnesota Symposium on Child Psychology. Developmental neuroscience. Volume 24*. Hillsdale, NJ: Lawrence Erlbaum; 1992.

5 Shore AN. The experience-dependent maturation of a regulatory system in the orbital prefrontal cortex and the origin of developmental psychopathology. *Dev Psychopathol*. 1996; **8**: 59–87.

6 Hughes DA. *Building the Bonds of Attachment: awakening love in deeply troubled children.* Nothvale, NJ: Jason Aronson Inc.; 1998.

7 Jackson G. *A Curious Consensus: 'brain scans prove disease?'*; http://psychrights.org/articles/GEJacksonMD BrainScanCuriousConsensus.pdf (accessed 22 July 2006).

8 Jackson G, ibid.

9 Leo J, Cohen D. Broken brains or flawed studies? A critical review of ADHD neuroimaging research. *J Mind Behav.* 2003; **24**: 29–56.

10 Castellanos FX, Lee PP, Sharp W *et al.* Developmental trajectories of brain volume abnormalities in children and adolescents with attention deficit hyperactivity disorder. *JAMA.* 2002; **288**: 1740–48.

11 Castellanos FX, cited by O'Meara KP. In ADHD studies, pictures may lie. *Insight on the News*, 19 August 2003.

12 Leo J, cited by O'Meara KP. In ADHD studies, pictures may lie. *Insight on the News*, 19 August 2003.

13 Cohen D. An update on ADHD neuroimaging research. *J Mind Behav.* 2004; **25**: 161–6.

14 Timimi S. *Naughty Boys.* Basingstoke: Palgrave Macmillan; 2005.

15 Maguire EA, Gadian DG, Johnsrude IS *et al.* Navigation-related structural change in the hippocampi of taxi drivers. *Proc Natl Acad Sci USA.* 2000; **97**: 4398–403.

16 Timimi S, op. cit.

17 Calvin W. *The Ascent of Mind.* New York: Bantam; 1990.

18 Ash T. *The Relationship Between the Mind and the Brain*; http://users.ox.ac.uk/~mert2049/philosophy/ash-mindandbrain.shtml (accessed 1 August 2006).

19 Schwartz JM, Stoessel PW, Baxter LR *et al.* Systematic changes in cerebral glucose metabolic rate after successful behaviour modification treatment of obsessive-compulsive disorder. *Arch Gen Psychiatry.* 1996; **53**: 109–13.

20 Leuchter AF, Cook LA, Witte EA. Changes in brain function of depressed patients during treatment with placebo. *Am J Psychiatry.* 2002; **159**: 122–9.

21 Timimi S, op. cit.

22 Flaherty LT, Arroyo W, Chatoor I *et al.* (2005) Brain Imaging and Child and Adolescent Psychiatry with special emphasis on SPECT. Retrieved by Grace Jackson on 9 July 2005, from www.psych.org/psych_pract?clin_issues/populations/children/SPECT.pdf; cited in Jackson GE. A Curious Consensus: 'brain scans prove disease?'; http://psychrights.org/articles/GEJacksonMDBrainScanCuriousConsensus.pdf (accessed 22 July 2006).

23 Jackson G, ibid.

Chapter 9

1 Baldwin S. Impact evaluation of a mass media public education campaign on clinic service provision for minors diagnosed with ADHD/ADD: audit survey of 100 index families. *Int J Risk Safety Med.* 2000; **13**: 203–19.

2 Sinclair S, Harris G. *ADHD clinics in East Staffordshire: survey findings.* Unpublished research.

3 Breggin P. *Toxic Psychiatry. Drugs and electroconvulsive therapy: the truth and the better alternatives.* London: Harper Collins; 1993.

4 Keirsey D. Private communication, 1988. Cited by Breggin P, op. cit.

5 Baldwin S. *When is an Amphetamine Not an Amphetamine?* www2.netdoctor.co.uk/editors_voice/index.asp?mode=showentry&entryId=50 (accessed 27 June 2006).

6 Jensen P, Bain M, Josephson A. *Why Johnny Can't Sit Still: kids' ideas on why they take stimulants.* Unpublished report.

7 Layard R. *Mental Health: Britain's biggest social problem?*; www.strategy.gov.uk/downloads/files/mh_layard.pdf (accessed 1 July 2006).

8 Breggin P, op. cit.

Chapter 10

1 Editorial. 'The big idea'. *BMJ.* 1996; **312**: 985.

2 Payne S. *Poverty and Social Exclusion Survey of Britain.* Bristol: Townsend Centre for International Poverty Research, University of Bristol; 2001.

3 Rogers A, Pilgrim D. *Mental Health and Inequality.* Basingstoke: Palgrave Macmillan; 2003.

4 Bertram M. www.psychminded.co.uk/news/news2003/july03/Social%20inequalities,%20madness%20and%20the%20system%20where%20are%20we.htm (accessed 22 July 2006).

5 Green H, McGinnity A, Meltzer H *et al. Mental Health of Children and Young People in Great Britain, 2004.* Basingstoke: Palgrave Macmillan; 2005.

6 Lerner MJ, Miller DT. Just World research and the attribution process: looking back and ahead. *Psychol Bull.* 1979; **85**: 1030–51.

7 Acheson D. *Independent Inquiry into Inequalities in Health Report.* London: The Stationery Office; 1998.

8 BBC World News. *Health Inequality Gap 'Widening'*, broadcast 11 August 2005; http://news.bbc.co.uk/2/hi/health/4139440.stm (accessed 2 July 2006).

9 Dorling D, cited on BBC World News, ibid.

10 Koivusalo M. The future of European health policies. *Int J Health Serv.* 2005; **35**: 325–42.

11 Koivusalo M, ibid.

12 Amicus. *Evidence to the Health Committee's Inquiry into NHS Deficits*; www.amicustheunion.org (accessed 1 August 2006).

13 Hallowell M. *What Problems Does PFI Present for Barts and the London NHS Trust?* Edinburgh: Centre for International Public Health Policy, University of Edinburgh; 2006.

14 Hallowell M, ibid.

15 Aldred R. *In the Interests of Profit, at the Expense of Patients: an examination of the NHS Local Improvement Finance Trust (LIFT) model, analysing six key disadvantages.* London: UNISON; 2006.

16 Bosanquet N, Haldenby A, de Zoete H. *Investment in the NHS: facing up to the reform agenda*; www.reform.co.uk/filestore/pdf/Investment%20in%20the%20NHS,%20Reform,%202006.pdf (accessed 2 August 2006).

17 Miller P. Speech to the BMA Consultants' Conference, 7 June 2006; www.bma.org.uk?ap.nsf/content/PaulMillerSpeechCCSCConf2006 (accessed 1 September 2006).

18 Miller P, ibid.

19 Miller P, ibid.

20 *Britain's Botched Operations: summary by Keep our NHS Public*; www.healthdemocracy.org.uk/healthdemocracy.org.uk/HealthPolicy/GovernmentPolicy/DiagnosticAndTreatmentCentres/Sources.htm (accessed 1 August 2006).

21 BBC News. *Private Treatment Centres Warning*, broadcast 15 December 2005. www.healthdemocracy.org.uk/healthdemocracy.org.uk/HealthPolicy/GovernmentPolicy/DiagnosticAndTreatmentCentres/Sources.htm (accessed 1 August 2006).

22 *NHS IT supplier iSoft in serious trouble – massive risk for NPFIT*; www.publictechnology. net (accessed 30 August 2006).
23 Jeffcott M, Johnson C. *The Use of a Formalised Risk Model in NHS Information System Development.* Glasgow: Department of Computer Science, University of Glasgow; 2002.
24 Miller P, op. cit.

Chapter 11

1 Southall A. What we have learned from working with children (or why we need a revolution in mental health). *Clin Psychol Forum.* 2006; **164**: 33–6.
2 House of Commons Health Committee. *The Influence of the Pharmaceutical Industry. Fourth Report of Session 2004–2005. Volume II. Formal minutes, oral and written evidence.* London: The Stationery Office; 2005.
3 Hall B. Pfizer ditched UK move due to tough planning laws. *The Financial Times*, 26 June 2006.
4 Blitz J. Brown in drive to streamline planning. *The Financial Times*, 3 July 2006.
5 House of Commons Health Committee, op. cit.
6 Dewey J. *Democracy and Education: An Introduction to the Philosophy of Education.* New York: Free Press; 1916. Cited by Beck J. *Writing the Radical Centre: William Carlos Williams, John Dewey and American cultural politics.* Albany, NY: SUNY Press; 2001.
7 House of Commons Health Committee, op. cit.
8 House of Commons Health Committee, op. cit.
9 Zaslow J. Do anti-ADHD drugs stifle creativity? *The Wall Street Journal*, 14 February 2005.
10 Chomsky N. Transcript of lecture, *'Control of Our Lives'*, delivered in the Kira Auditorium, Albuquerque, New Mexico, 26 February 2000; www.zmag.org/ chomskyalbuq.htm (accessed 1 August 2006).

Appendix 1

1 The MTA Cooperative Group. A 14-month randomized clinical trial of treatment strategies for attention-deficit/hyperactivity disorder. Multimodal Treatment Study of Children with ADHD. *Arch Gen Psychiatry.* 1999; **56**(12): 1073–86.
2 Breggin PR. A critical analysis of the NIMH Multimodal Treatment Study for attention-deficit/hyperactivity disorder (The MTA Study). Available at www.breggin.com/mta. html (accessed 12 February 2005).

Index

3